How Your Baby Is Born

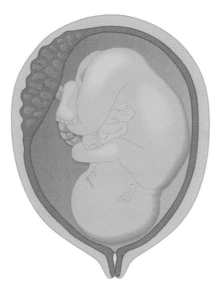

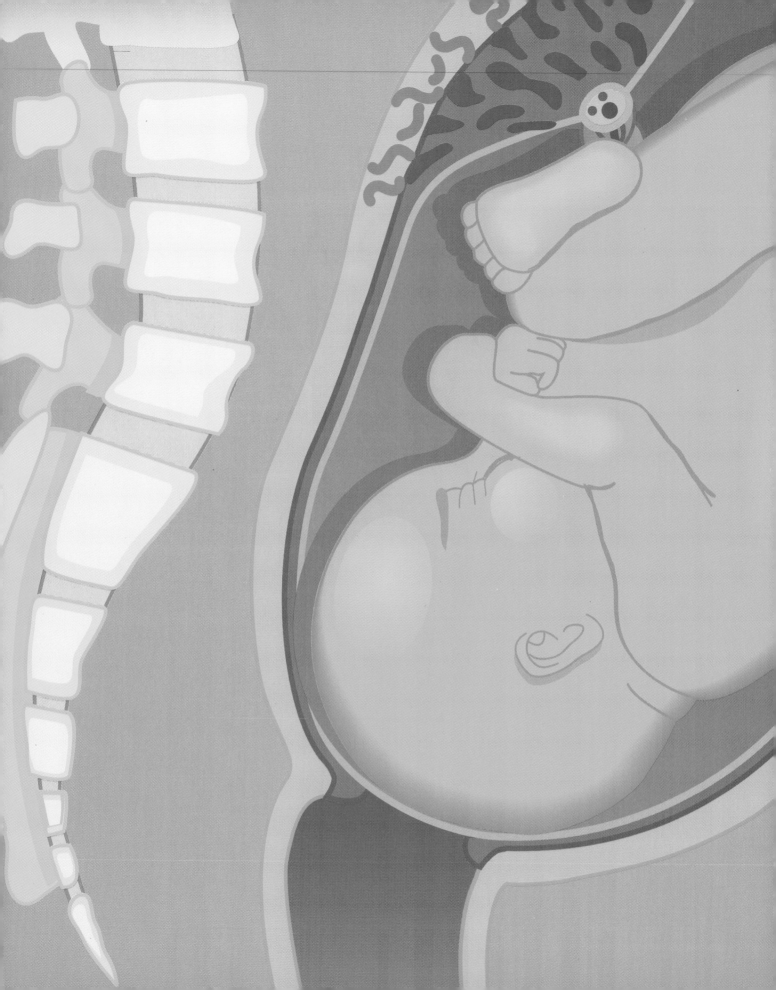

HOW YOUR BABY IS BORN

AMY B. TUTEUR, M.D.

Illustrated by
FRAN MILNER AND TERRY TOYAMA

Ziff-Davis Press
Emeryville, California

Development Editor	Valerie Haynes Perry
Copy Editor	Kayla Sussell
Technical Reviewer	Rima Goldman, M.D.
Project Coordinator	Cort Day
Proofreader	Carol Burbo
Cover Illustration	Fran Milner and Terry Toyama
Cover Design	Regan Honda
Book Design	Carrie English
Technical Illustration	Fran Milner and Terry Toyama
Word Processing	Howard Blechman
Page Layout	Tony Jonick
Indexer	Anne Leach

Ziff-Davis Press books are produced on a Macintosh computer system with the following applications: FrameMaker®, Microsoft® Word, QuarkXPress®, Adobe Illustrator®, Adobe Photoshop®, Adobe Streamline™, MacLink®*Plus*, Aldus® FreeHand™, Collage Plus™.

If you have comments or questions or would like to receive a free catalog, call or write:
Ziff-Davis Press
5903 Christie Avenue
Emeryville, CA 94608
1-800-688-0448

ISBN 1-56276-239-7

Manufactured in the United States of America
⊕ This book is printed on paper that contains 50% total recycled fiber of which 20% is de-inked postconsumer fiber.
10 9 8 7 6 5 4 3 2

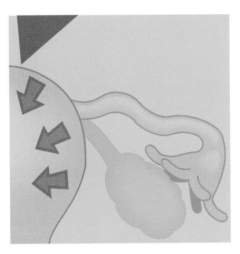

For my babies, Alex, David, Jeffrey,
and their sibling to be

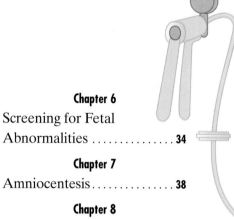

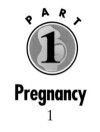

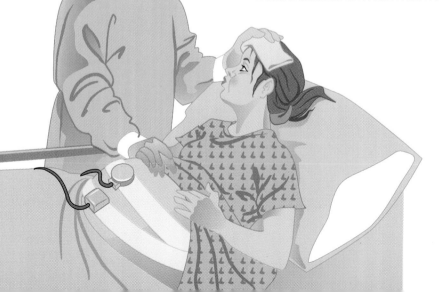

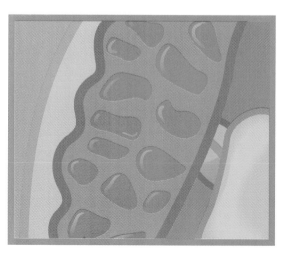

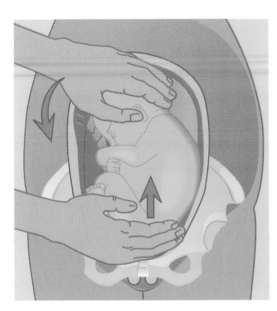

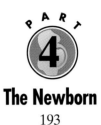

P A R T

4

The Newborn
193

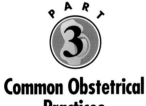

P A R T

3

Common Obstetrical Practices
117

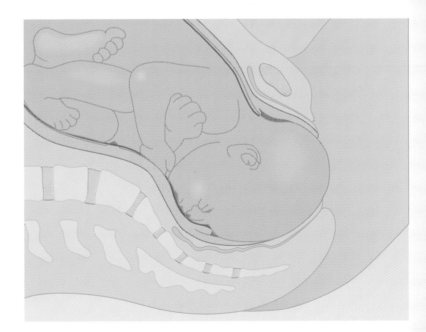

This book, like a baby, took nine months to grow and develop. However, unlike my children, which my husband and I created as a relatively simple at-home project, *How Your Baby Is Born* required the cross-country collaboration of many people.

I would like to thank the many individuals at Ziff-Davis Press who gave their time and effort unstintingly. Thanks to Cindy Hudson, who believed in the project from the start. Thanks to Eric Stone for advice and encouragement along the way. A big, big thank-you to Valerie Haynes Perry for her invaluable editing, which was always gentle, but firm. Thanks to Kayla Sussell, Rima Goldman, M.D., and Cort Day, all of whom provided technical and editorial input. A special thank-you to Fran Milner and Terry Toyama who created the magnificent artwork in the book. Their achievement is all the more remarkable when you consider that they started with sketches that I submitted filled with stick-figure babies growing inside stick-figure mothers.

Thanks to my friends and colleagues including Susan Wilcove; Joyce Kozol; Cindy Gray; Linda Leviel, C.N.M.; Sibel Bessim, M.D.; and Vanessa Barss, M.D. They each read portions of the manuscript and provided valuable feedback.

An obstetrician is made, not born. Thank you to the nurses and doctors of the Beth Israel Hospital in Boston who trained me. I also wish to thank the midwives, nurses, and doctors of the Brigham and Women's Hospital and Harvard Community Health Plan who are my colleagues and companions in a collaborative effort to deliver healthy babies to healthy mothers. I extend my deepest gratitude to the thousands of patients and their families who have allowed me to share the intimate moment of birth. From them, I have learned a great deal about the personal experience of childbirth as well as the process.

Finally, and most importantly, thank you to my husband Michael, who has read and commented on every word in this book. He has been by my side through medical school, residency, the births of three children (soon to be four), and the building of one house. You know it's really true love when you can let your husband edit your writing!

Some people always bring along a travel guide when they go on a trip. They pore over the maps, study the local customs, and try to learn a bit of the native language. This additional knowledge makes their trip both more comfortable and more enjoyable.

You can think of *How Your Baby Is Born* as your travel guide on your journey through the process of birth. Although the distance is short—just a few inches from inside your uterus to the outside world and into your arms—the trip you take with your baby is indeed a new and wondrous journey. Like a travel guide, *How Your Baby Is Born* offers you detailed maps, an introduction to the local customs, and a smattering of the native tongue. In this book, the color illustrations are your maps; you will learn about the local customs and procedures that are related to your visits to the hospital; and you will be able to add terms like *amniocentesis* and *placenta* to your vocabulary.

Read this book before you visit with your practitioner. Take it with you to your doctor's or midwife's office and use the illustrations to enhance his or her explanations. In fact, your doctor might find the illustrations a helpful aid in answering your questions. Take this book with you to the hospital or birthing center so that the new place won't seem strange or frightening. Use it to help you make the decisions you need to make to help ensure the kind of birth experience that you hope to have.

Like a traditional travel guide, the goal of this book is to help you feel less foreign and more familiar with new surroundings and the new experiences of pregnancy, labor, and delivery. You should know what the amniocentesis procedure will be like before you have one done. If your baby is breech, you should understand what that means and not become alarmed by the term. When you walk into the hospital birthing room, you should recognize the various pieces of equipment and what they are used for. Above all, you should feel neither frightened nor threatened by the new environment and experiences.

And, just as a travel guide cannot tell you exactly what you should see or do to have the best possible trip, this book cannot tell you what you must do to have the best possible birth experience. That's because, like a trip itinerary, what's great for one person may be disappointing for another. Your journey toward becoming a parent is a deeply personal one. Use this book to understand your options and explore your preferences. Do you wish to minimize intervention during labor and delivery, or do the high-tech tools and equipment of the modern hospital provide you with a sense of security during an anxiety-provoking time? Use this book to decide what a good birth experience means to you. Then, don't hesitate to share your preferences with your obstetrician or midwife. Your practitioner will not know what you want unless you discuss it beforehand.

Unlike a traditional travel guide, this one intends that everyone winds up at exactly the same place: with a healthy baby and a healthy mother. Most of the time, no special effort is required to reach this outcome. Unfortunately, we cannot predict which labors might be difficult or which babies might not easily withstand the strain. Above all, be flexible. It might turn out that your baby needs more intervention than you would have wished. That can be a disappointment, but may be less of one if you keep in mind that your deepest wish is for a healthy child.

How Your Baby Is Born covers the following four territories: Pregnancy, Labor and Delivery, Common Obstetrical Procedures, and The Newborn. While the organization within each section is chronological, it is not necessary to read the chapters in a sequential order. Each chapter is a self-contained discussion of a topic that does not rely on information that is covered elsewhere in the book.

This book does not contain every possible situation encountered in pregnancy, nor is every possible obstetrical procedure described. Because mastering the practice of obstetrics takes many years of study and experience, no single book could encompass the entire subject.

The information in this book is not intended to substitute for consultation with your own obstetrician or midwife. You can compare reading *How Your Baby Is Born* to working with an experienced travel agent in planning a lengthy and extensive excursion. Each pregnancy, labor, and delivery is unique, just as each baby is unique. Only someone familiar with every detail of your situation is qualified to make recommendations about your obstetrical management. However, this book will provide you with detailed explanations of the most commonly encountered issues and obstetrical practices, which will allow you to participate as a full partner in any decision making that may be required.

The ultimate goal of a travel guide is to make your trip as easy and as enjoyable as it can be. *How Your Baby Is Born* shares this goal. Giving birth to a new life is nothing short of a miracle. Enjoy your part in this miracle to the fullest and celebrate your role in creating and nurturing the new life within you. Prepare to bring your child forth to share in the excitement of your world and the security of your love.

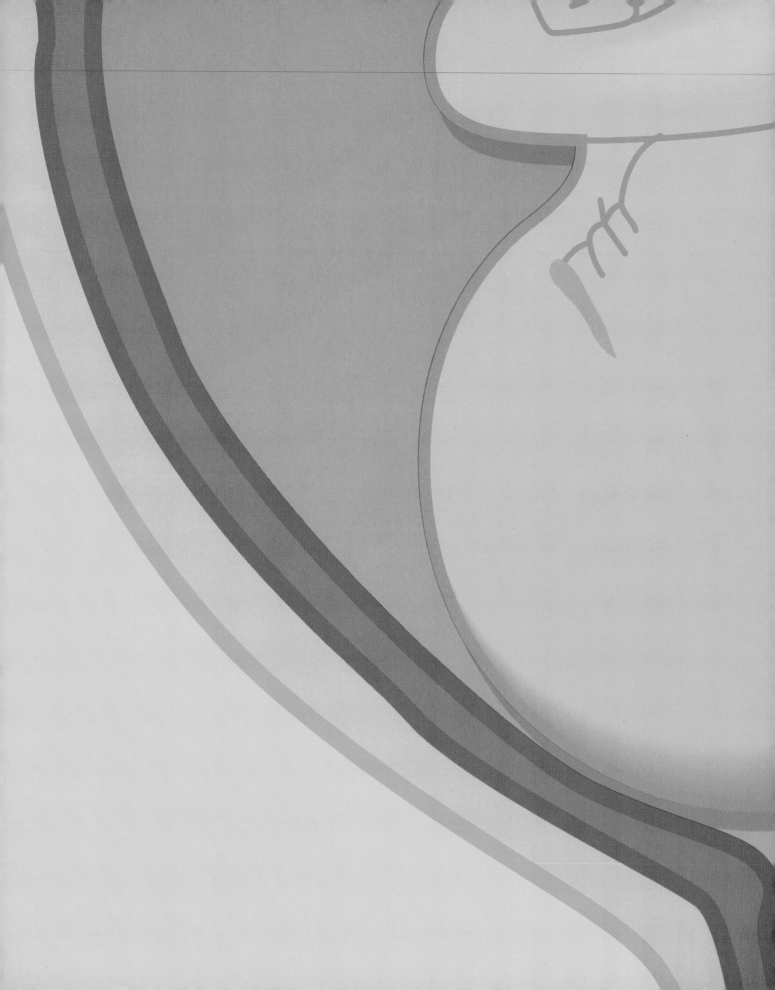

PREGNANCY

CONTENTS

O V E R V I E W

Congratulations! You're expecting a baby! You may be excited, surprised, nervous, or a bit of all three. Your thoughts skip ahead to the day you'll hold your new baby in your arms. You anticipate choosing baby furniture and planning your delivery. And, in the 1990s, there are so many delivery options available, you can often plan the type of delivery that you would like to have. But before you jump ahead to the main event, there are a few decisions that you will need to make during your pregnancy.

This section covers the course of normal pregnancy, routine prenatal tests, and some advanced technology. How does your baby develop? What changes does your body undergo during pregnancy? Chapters 1, 2, and 3 are devoted to the basic facts and terms used in discussing pregnancy.

Why should you routinely visit your obstetrician or midwife? What will happen during these prenatal visits? Chapters 4 and 5 explain how your pregnancy will be monitored. You'll learn about the measurements and testing that occur during the visits to your obstetrician or midwife. The routine tests you'll take during your pregnancy are discussed, as well as more advanced tests that are used in the event that potential problems are detected. For example, Chapters 6 and 7 discuss alphafetoprotein (AFP) tests and amniocentesis. The AFP assay can detect abnormalities by measuring concentrations of certain hormones in the mother's blood. Amniocentesis is the process by which the fetal chromosomes are directly analyzed.

Fortunately, most pregnancies proceed without problems. However, it's good to be prepared if you should encounter difficulties. Chapters 8, 9, and 10 offer an in-depth discussion of common problems in pregnancy. These chapters also cover diagnosis and treatment.

Any type of medical test can be anxiety provoking, but when you understand the purpose and method of testing, you may worry less. During pregnancy, two types of tests can be performed. These are screening tests and diagnostic tests. Screening tests are ordered routinely. They have been designed to be used on a large population to detect the *possible* presence of problems. The results are analyzed by comparing your test value to that of everyone in the large population. If your results are significantly different than average, it is possible that you may be affected by the problem the screening test was designed to detect. If this is the case, a diagnostic test will be recommended to determine whether you are truly affected.

Screening tests are designed in such a way that they err on the side of over diagnosis rather than under diagnosis. This means many more women will be asked to take diagnostic tests than will ultimately be found to have the condition under consideration. This is deliberate because testing more people than necessary is a precaution against missing someone who needs treatment. In practical terms, it means you should not be alarmed if the results of any of your screening tests are abnormal. The odds are still high that no problem exists. Of course, asking a pregnant woman not to worry is like asking her not to breathe—it's practically impossible.

If your practitioner suspects a problem, he or she will order diagnostic tests. The results of these tests can actually constitute a diagnosis. Such tests include ultrasound, which allow a partial visualization of the developing baby, and amniocentesis. Blood tests for determining glucose concentration to rule out gestational diabetes (diabetes of pregnancy) are another example of a commonly administered diagnostic test.

You may wonder why you should even bother with any prenatal testing. After all, pregnancy is now widely thought to be virtually risk free for mother and baby. You may even hear some people say that pregnancy and childbirth are "natural events," implying that nothing can go wrong. It's important to remember, though, that pregnancy-related problems are "natural," too. In fact, up until this century, pregnancy was considered quite dangerous for both mother and baby. The difference now is that we monitor pregnant women very carefully for any pregnancy-related problems. And we are better able to deal with many of these problems very early, before they can cause harm either to the mother or the baby.

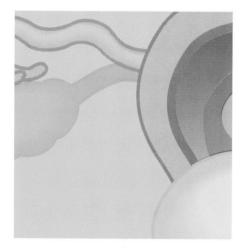

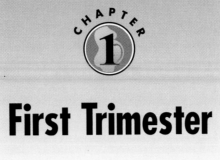

First Trimester

THE FIRST TRIMESTER includes the pre-embryonic period and encompasses weeks three through ten. You might wonder what happened to weeks one and two. Pregnancies are conventionally dated with reference to the woman's last menstrual period. That's because most women don't know when conception actually occurred, but they can usually remember the first day of their last period.

The due date is calculated by adding 280 days (40 weeks) to the date of the first day of the last menstrual period. Obstetricians and midwives don't actually do the addition, of course. They use a *pregnancy wheel*, a plastic or cardboard wheel that is designed to show the date 40 weeks from any date on the calendar. The due date is not absolute: Only 16 percent of babies are actually born on the due date. The vast majority of babies is born between 38 and 42 weeks.

During the first trimester, most of the action takes place on the inside, and what a lot of action there is. You don't automatically look pregnant, and initially you might not even feel pregnant. But you are very likely to develop a lot of symptoms that are the result of the pregnancy. That's because the developing placenta produces hormones that have a variety of effects on maternal organs. For example, during the first trimester, the placenta produces hormones that already begin acting on the breasts in preparation for breast-feeding. Increased breast growth occurs that can cause temporary breast tenderness. And everyone knows about pregnancy-induced nausea ("morning sickness"), but tiredness and weight gain are also very common. You may even notice that your hair looks better when you're pregnant. Because of the increased blood flow associated with pregnancy, hair grows faster and thicker. Unfortunately, after delivery, things return to normal.

The baby undergoes its most complex and important stage of growth during the first trimester. In fact, a human being grows faster during this period than at any other time in pregnancy, childhood, or puberty. The fertilized egg divides repeatedly, and the resulting cells organize into the embryo and the placenta. By week 12, all external structures and internal organs have been formed. The embryo is easily recognizable as human and has begun moving freely within the amniotic sac. Over the next 28 weeks the fetus grows and the organ systems mature, but no new structures develop.

First Trimester: The Embryo in Utero

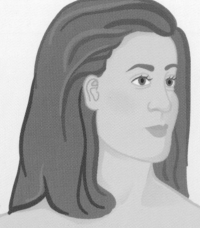

Ovary In the early weeks, the ovary produces hormones that support the pregnancy. The site that releases the ovum becomes the *corpus luteum*, a tiny hormone factory that supplies the mother with the necessary hormones until the placenta can take over. The corpus luteum can grow in size to become a cyst on the ovary and is often seen on ultrasounds done in the first trimester. This is a normal finding and should not cause concern.

GI tract The hormones that are produced during pregnancy affect the digestive system. Side effects are not limited to "morning sickness," but may also include bloating, constipation, and (as the baby grows) heartburn.

Uterus The embryo is protected in the amniotic sac within the uterus. Although the embryo is only slightly more than two inches long, all external structures and internal organs are present.

Bladder Notice how close the uterus is to the bladder. This is why pregnant women have an increased urge to urinate—the growing uterus actually presses on the bladder.

Placenta   The placenta develops along with the embryo. In addition to extracting oxygen and nutrients from the mother's bloodstream, the placenta produces hormones that support the pregnancy. Among the first hormones that the placenta produces is *human chorionic gonadotropin* (HCG). This is the hormone that is measured by the blood tests that determine pregnancy. It is possible to diagnose pregnancy by a blood test even before the first day of the mother's period would be due. No HCG is detectable in the mother's blood-stream until implantation of the fertilized egg has occurred. Urine pregnancy tests also measure HCG. However, they are less sensitive than the blood test and cannot detect a preg-nancy until the day of the missed period.

Uterine wall   The uterus enlarges to accommodate the advancing pregnancy. In addition, the muscle of the uterine wall begins to grow thicker in preparation for the labor contractions required to push the baby out during delivery.

Embryo   Although the embryo must be enlarged to several times its actual size to see the details, it is ap-parent that all external structures are formed. However, notice that the body proportions are very different from those of chil-dren or adults. For example, an em-bryo's head is much larger in relation to its body than is a child's or an adult's.

Amniotic fluid   The embryo is cushioned and protected by the am-niotic fluid. At this stage, the volume of amniotic fluid is relatively large compared to embryonic size. That leaves lots of room for the embryo to move around. During the first trimester, the embryo is less likely to contact the uterine wall and be perceived by the mother than in the second and third trimesters.

PREGNANCY CALCULATOR

January February March April May December November October

LMP

Urine Pregnancy Test Positive

Weeks AVG. FETAL WT.-GRAMS AVG. FETAL LENGTH-CM

Probable Day of Conception

First day of Last menstrual Period

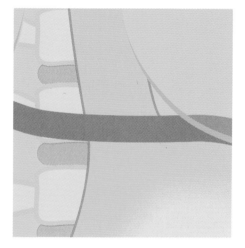

Second Trimester

MANY WOMEN CONSIDER the second trimester (weeks 13 through 26) the best part of pregnancy. Here's why: The symptoms of the first few months have largely abated, and the discomforts of the last trimester have not yet started.

Now your pregnancy is visible for all the world to see! If you have not already started to wear maternity clothes, you'll likely need them now. Each week your developing baby—now officially a fetus—grows a bit more. Your practitioner will measure fetal growth at your prenatal visits, albeit indirectly. He or she will use a tape measure to determine the distance from your pubic bone to the top of the uterus (also known as the *fundus*). This measurement is known as the fundal height.

During the second trimester, the mother first notices fetal movement, generally some time between 16–20 weeks. However, reflexive movements begin during the embryonic period, and the fetus becomes active before the mother notices. Early in pregnancy, the fetal movements are relatively weak, and there is a greater amount of room available for movement. Therefore, it is unlikely that the fetus will bang up against the uterine wall with enough force for Mom to notice.

Experienced mothers remember the first flutterings from previous pregnancies and are more attuned to even the weakest movements. That's why they are more likely to notice fetal movement earlier. Later in pregnancy, the fetus is much stronger and relatively more confined. In fact, fetal movements become so vigorous they can be observed through the mother's abdominal wall. They have been known to keep expectant mothers up half the night—and expectant fathers, too, if the parents-to-be sleep too close together!

Vital organs continue to mature throughout the second trimester. Babies born before approximately 24 weeks are considered pre-viable (too young to survive). That's because their lungs are not sufficiently developed to exchange oxygen. The lungs gradually begin to acquire this critical capacity during the last several weeks of the second trimester. However, with appropriate support in a neonatal intensive care unit, most babies born after 26 weeks can survive. Babies born at this early age may weigh as little as two pounds and may have extremely serious medical problems.

The development of the external genitalia is completed early in the second trimester, and the baby's sex can usually be recognized by ultrasound at the same time that it is safe to perform amniocentesis. In females, the fetal ovary undergoes significant development during the second trimester. Remarkably, all the ova that the ovaries will ever contain are formed by the fifth month of fetal life! After their formation, the ova enter a state of rest in which they will remain until puberty. Nature prepares for the next generation even before the new generation is born!

Several important prenatal tests are administered during the second trimester. These include ultrasound, serum alphafetoprotein assay (AFP), and, possibly, amniocentesis. These tests will be covered in Chapters 4, 6, and 7.

Second Trimester: The Fetus in Utero

As the abdominal cavity becomes more crowded, pressure is exerted upward on the diaphragm, making it harder to take a deep breath. This restriction on the lungs, coupled with the increased oxygen requirement of the developing fetus, is responsible for the shortness of breath that pregnant women often experience with even minor exertion.

The mother's center of gravity changes as the uterus grows. To accommodate this change and allow the mother to balance properly, the spine develops a more prominent curve known as a *lordosis*. Lordosis accounts for the typical posture a woman assumes during pregnancy.

As the uterus grows out of the pelvis, it stretches the round ligaments that normally hold it in position. You can see the ligaments here. The stretching of these ligaments produces round ligament pain, another common complaint associated with the second trimester. *Round ligament pain* is sudden, sharp pain in the lower abdomen on one or both sides of the uterus. The pain often occurs when the mother moves, and it goes away spontaneously. It is not harmful in any way to the mother or baby.

The uterus has grown out of the pelvis and into the abdominal cavity. Now, it displaces the abdominal organs; this leads to one of the most common complaints of pregnancy—heartburn.

The *placenta* is well developed now. It is truly an amazing organ. The placenta develops as the baby does, from cells derived from the original cell formed by the union of the ovum and sperm. It is a part of the baby—the part that is destined to be jettisoned at the time of delivery. The placenta mediates between fetal circulation and maternal circulation, allowing the fetus to extract oxygen and nutrients from the mother's bloodstream. The fetus also passes its waste products across the placenta so that they can be excreted by the mother. Finally, the placenta produces hormones that primarily affect the mother, helping her body support the pregnancy and prepare for delivery, and even for future breast-feeding.

The skin is thin and wrinkled now, but fat deposition is beginning. The sebaceous glands of the fetal skin begin producing vernix during the second trimester. *Vernix* is a thick, white, fatty substance; it looks and acts like cold cream and protects fetal skin from the constant exposure to amniotic fluid.

Notice that the fetus still has lots of room to move around. The positions it favors during the second trimester have no bearing on whether it will be facing head down, as it should, at the time of delivery.

During the latter part of the second trimester, the eyelids become fully developed, and the fetus can open his or her eyes. The eyebrows are also well developed, but the eyelashes won't appear for a few more weeks.

The fingernails are present by the end of the second trimester. At the rate that the new fingernails grow, they should just reach the tips of the fingers by the time of birth. Babies that are born more than a week or two after their due date have fingernails that are too long, and they may have scratched themselves before birth.

Amniotic fluid is, in large part, fetal urine. It is produced by the fetal kidneys, but unlike normal urine, it does not contain waste products. (Fetal wastes are eliminated by transfer across the placenta to the mother's bloodstream.) During the second trimester, the volume of amniotic fluid increases considerably, and it becomes safe to remove a small amount by *amniocentesis*. This procedure is done because the amniotic fluid contains skin cells that the fetus has shed. They can be analyzed to determine whether the fetus has any chromosomal abnormalities.

Fetal blood travels to the placenta and back to the fetus through the umbilical cord, which contains two umbilical arteries and one umbilical vein. Deoxygenated blood that has been returned to the fetal heart is sent out to the placenta through the umbilical arteries; oxygenated blood travels through the umbilical vein back to the heart, where it is distributed to the rest of the fetal circulation. Some important differences exist between fetal circulation and newborn circulation. And amazingly, the transition between the two types of circulation occurs almost completely at the moment that the newborn draws his or her first breath (see Chapter 28 for more on this).

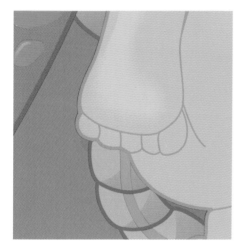

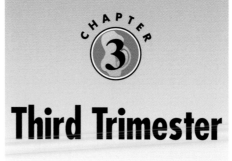

Third Trimester

PREGNANCY IS A "low glamour" state, and at no time is this more apparent than in the third trimester (weeks 27 through 40). Everyone asks you how you feel, and you feel great, except for (choose one or more from the following list): heartburn, hemorrhoids, constipation, varicose veins, backache, difficulty sleeping, and the urge to urinate every half hour!

Most of these discomforts are the result of your baby's increasing size. But this continued growth is responsible for exciting developments as well. The fetus moves in a regular pattern each day, and many expectant women get to know their babies' characteristic movements. You need never feel alone; you always have your "buddy" with you.

Prenatal visits should become more frequent in the third trimester, increasing from once every four weeks to every other week. During the last month of pregnancy, you should visit your practitioner once a week. The increasing frequency of visits allows your doctor or midwife to monitor you and your baby more closely for some common complications of pregnancy, including pre-eclampsia (covered in Chapter 10), premature labor, and gestational diabetes.

If there are any concerns about fetal growth, your practitioner will probably order an ultrasound test (covered in the next chapter). If the fundal height is less than expected, you may not be as far along as you thought (perhaps you miscalculated the first day of your last period). If there is other evidence that confirms the gestational age (an earlier ultrasound, or previous exams that were consistent with your original due date), there is a possibility that the baby is not growing properly. An ultrasound exam can determine gestational age as well as fetal size, and thereby explain why the baby may be smaller than anticipated.

If the fundal height is greater than expected, there are other reasons why the fetal size might be greater than gestational age would indicate, including multiple pregnancy (twins, triplets or more) and *polyhydramnios* (excess amniotic fluid). Once again, ultrasound is the test of choice to further evaluate the discrepancy. However, it is important to remember that in most situations in which an ultrasound is ordered to evaluate fundal heights that are less than or greater than gestational age, nothing is wrong. In those cases, the discrepancy probably represents individual variation. After all, not all babies weigh the same when they are born.

As the third trimester progresses, you'll probably feel increasing excitement (and possibly a bit of apprehension) about your impending labor and delivery. The uterus offers gentle reminders in the form of *Braxton-Hicks contractions*. These are weak uterine contractions that generally become noticeable in the third trimester. They are normal and can be distinguished from labor contractions in a number of ways. First, they are generally very mild, causing a sensation of "tightening," without pain. Second, they do not develop any regular pattern. Third, they do not become progressively more frequent or more painful; they just go away. It's almost as if the uterus is practicing for the labor ahead.

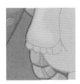

Third Trimester: The Fetus in Utero

During the third trimester (and sometimes even earlier), the mother's breasts begin to produce colostrum. *Colostrum* is the "pre-milk" secreted at the end of pregnancy. It is different from the milk that comes later and is very rich in antibodies. These antibodies can provide the newborn temporary protection from many illnesses to which the mother is already immune. Colostrum can be clear, white, or yellow. It may leak from the breast spontaneously, or may be released by massaging the nipple and *areola*, the dark area around the nipple.

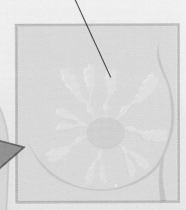

The placenta continues to supply the fetus with oxygen and nutrients. As the due date approaches, and particularly after the due date has passed, the placenta may become less successful in meeting all the baby's needs. This may be because the baby is so large that it outstrips the placenta's capacity, or it may result from the placenta just being "old." The placenta doesn't seem to function as well once the due date is a week or two past. Diminished placental capacity may cause decreased fetal growth and decreased fetal ability to tolerate labor. For these reasons, a pregnancy should not be allowed to continue more than two weeks past the due date; labor should be induced if that date is reached.

Tremendous growth takes place during the third trimester. The baby's weight increases from about 2 pounds to the delivery weight, which can be anywhere from 6 to 9 pounds. The average newborn weighs approximately 7 pounds, but a few babies weigh less than 6 pounds, and some weigh more than 10 pounds.

There is approximately one quart of amniotic fluid now. If an ultrasound is done during the third trimester, the amount of amniotic fluid is assessed. If it is smaller than expected, it may be a subtle sign that the placenta is no longer functioning as well as possible.

The testicles in a male fetus develop in the abdomen and descend into the scrotum during the third trimester. Some premature babies are born with undescended testicles. They usually descend during the first few weeks of the baby's life outside of the womb.

Fetal lung maturity is attained during the third trimester. The baby's lungs begin to manufacture several substances critical to a newborn's respiration. These substances are released into the amniotic fluid and can be assessed by laboratory tests. If there is a need to deliver your baby prematurely, or if premature labor seems likely to cause a premature delivery, your practitioner can determine whether your baby's lungs have matured. This is done by testing a sample of the amniotic fluid obtained either by amniocentesis (the same procedure done for genetic analysis in the second trimester), or, if the membranes have ruptured, the fluid can be collected from the vagina.

During the third trimester, the fetal intestine begins producing *meconium*, which is made up of fetal wastes that cannot be removed across the maternal circulation. The meconium is expelled as the newborn's first few bowel movements. In cases of fetal distress during labor, the meconium may be expelled into the amniotic fluid, causing it to turn green. The presence of meconium-stained amniotic fluid during labor calls for increased vigilance.

An ultrasound done during the third trimester can produce a lot of information about the fetus. The ultrasound can determine the fetal size and position, and a biophysical profile can assess fetal well-being. The *biophysical profile* is a rating system for four different characteristics: fetal tone, fetal movement, amniotic fluid volume, and fetal breathing movements. For each parameter, a score ranging from 0 (abnormal) to 2 (normal) is given. A good score on the biophysical profile indicates a fetus whose placenta is supplying adequate amounts of oxygen and nutrients. A low score raises the possibility that the placenta may no longer be serving the fetus adequately. When combined with electronic monitoring of the fetal heart, the biophysical profile offers valuable information about the baby's well-being.

The uterus has to enlarge to 1,000 times its pre-pregnancy capacity! Amazingly, it will return to normal size within six weeks after delivery.

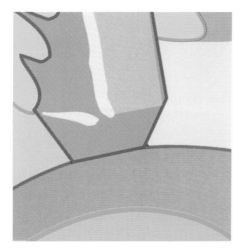

CHAPTER
4

Assessing the Baby

VISITING THE OBSTETRICIAN or midwife is the only medical appointment that many people actually enjoy. Each appointment is an opportunity to appreciate that the small, day-to-day changes have actually wrought great progress over the course of a month. It may seem that the obstetrical appointment is little more than a social engagement, with lots of conversation and very little obstetrical practice. However, with a few simple measurements, a lot of information can be gleaned about your developing baby's health.

Your practitioner starts each visit with questions about the baby's progress, and your pediatrician will do the same in the future. Have you felt the baby move yet? Most women expecting their first baby will notice fetal movement sometime after the 16th week, possibly not until the 20th week. Many women who have already delivered a child may perceive fetal movement even earlier.

The baby is also measured indirectly by measuring the fundal height, as mentioned in Chapter 2. The measurement of fundal height, in centimeters, normally corresponds to the age of the pregnancy, measured in weeks from the last menstrual period. So if you're twenty weeks pregnant, your fundal height should be approximately 20 centimeters (cm.).

Finally, the baby is evaluated by placing a doptone (see the first illustration in this chapter) on the mother's abdomen to listen for the baby's heartbeat. The *doptone* uses sound waves to sense the movement of the fetal heart and produces an audible beating sound that mimics the heart rate. The fetal heart rate should be between 120–160 beats per minute, although it may go higher for brief periods when the baby moves.

As you might imagine, though, the best way to assess the baby's health is to see the baby, and this can be done even before the baby is born, using ultrasound technology. Not only can the baby be measured and its weight calculated from those measurements, its internal anatomy also can be evaluated.

Ultrasound uses sound waves to create an image of the baby and its internal structures. The transducer (the instrument placed on the mother's abdomen) both emits and retrieves sound waves. By analyzing the changes that occur in the returning sound waves, a computerized reconstruction of the baby's anatomy can be created.

Ultrasound does not use radiation. The best studies to date indicate that ultrasound has no negative effects on either mother or baby. Nonetheless, ultrasound should be reserved only for answering medical questions, not for determining the baby's sex, or obtaining a picture for the new baby album. Although an ultrasound test can yield valuable information about individual babies, there is no evidence that routine ultrasound screening promotes better outcomes.

Ultrasound is completely painless, and actually lots of fun. If you're going to have an ultrasound test, you may want to bring Dad along as well. It's quite a thrill to see an image of your baby (even if it appears a bit skeletal), to watch the baby move, and possibly to see it suck its thumb.

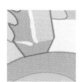

Monitoring the Baby's Heart

The doptone uses sound waves to sense the movement of the fetal heart. Some say it sounds like galloping horses' hooves.

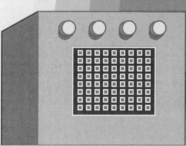

Doptone

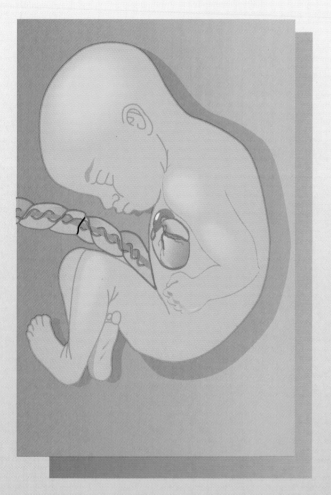

The doptone detects the motion of the fetal heart. It can "hear" the fetal heart only if it is properly positioned over it. That can be an especially tricky task in the second trimester, when the fetus has lots of room to move and can change position easily. The fetal heart is "heard" best through the baby's back. That means the baby's heart may be impossible to detect if his or her back is positioned against the mother's back. However, a little patience usually results in a position change, and then the heart rate can be determined.

In the third trimester, the location on the mother's abdomen where the fetal heart is best detected provides other, valuable information. If the baby is head down, his or her heart should be located below the level of the mother's navel. If your practitioner detects your baby's heartbeat above the level of your navel, it may indicate that your baby is in the breech position. Before 36 weeks, the baby's position is not important; he or she still has plenty of time and room to change to a head-first position.

An Ultrasound Exam in Progress

The ultrasound test is a painless procedure. You lie on an examining table and the technician puts ultrasound gel on your abdomen. (Ultrasound will not work if the sound waves travel through air, and the gel creates an air-free space between the transducer and your skin.) Your practitioner places the transducer on your abdomen, and the show begins.

The ultrasound machine is an incredible piece of technology. It analyzes the sound waves returning to the transducer from the fetus and compares them with the sound waves that were originally emitted. Discrepancies in the sound waves result when the soundwaves bounce off the internal structures of both the mother's body and the fetus, which lie underneath the transducer. This is how an image of these structures is generated.

Ultrasound doesn't just create a picture, it creates a video! Of course, it takes a little guidance to understand what you're looking at. With some help, you'll be able to discern your baby moving around—you'll see his or her face, and fingers, and even the beating heart.

Ultrasound gel

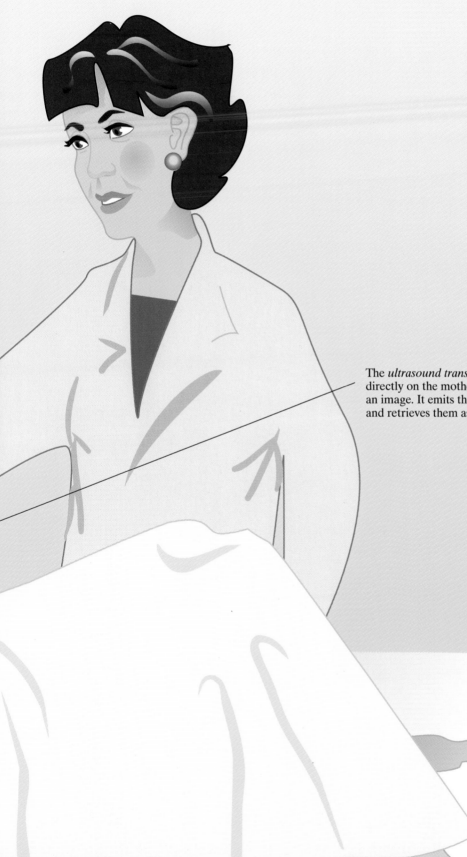

The *ultrasound transducer* must be placed directly on the mother's abdomen to obtain an image. It emits the ultrasound waves and retrieves them as they bounce back.

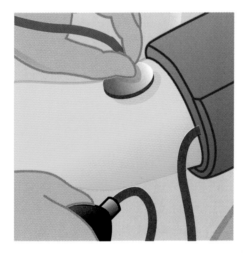

CHAPTER 5

Assessing the Mother

AT EVERY OBSTETRICAL visit, three aspects of your health are always measured. You are weighed, your blood pressure is checked, and your urine is tested for the amount of sugar and protein it contains. Why are these measurements so important?

Maternal weight provides both general and specific information. Good weight gain is usually associated with good fetal growth. You may find it hard to accept the idea that gaining weight is not only anticipated, it is also appreciated. You should not worry about a weight gain of 30 pounds or more. Remember, pregnancy is no time for dieting. However, in general, maternal weight gain should not exceed 40 pounds.

Checking your weight gain is helpful for monitoring excess fluid retention, which is a possible warning sign of pre-eclampsia. *Pre-eclampsia* (also known as toxemia or pregnancy-induced hypertension) is a disease of pregnancy. It is most common among women who are pregnant for the first time, and no one understand what causes it. Pre-eclampsia is characterized by high blood pressure, *edema* (swelling due to excess fluid retention) and protein in the urine. It can also be associated with other, even more serious problems. Fortunately, it can be effectively treated in the short term with medications, and reliably cured by delivering the baby. See Chapter 10 for details on pre-eclampsia.

The incidence of these symptoms explains the importance of the blood-pressure check and the urine assays (an *assay* is a test). Elevated blood pressure and the presence of protein in the urine are both early signs of pre-eclampsia. If these signs are present, your doctor or midwife can advise specific measures to lower your blood pressure and monitor you for signs of advancing illness. In most cases, bed rest can help control blood pressure elevation. Some cases of pre-eclampsia may require inducing labor before it begins spontaneously, often with no need for medication. Serious cases may require speicalized medication and other intervention. See Chapter 10 for details.

The medical assistant also evaluates your urine for the presence of glucose (sugar) in order to diagnose another pregnancy-related condition, *gestational diabetes*. Like other forms of diabetes, gestational diabetes affects the body's ability to process sugar. This form of diabetes results from the effect of pregnancy hormones on glucose metabolism, but it is completely reversed after delivery. Modification of the mother's diet can usually manage most cases of gestational diabetes. Insulin is rarely required. However, measuring the glucose in the mother's urine is a very imprecise diagnostic tool. Measuring the concentration of glucose in the mother's blood after she has drunk a sugary drink is a far better test. This is known as the glucose tolerance test, or the one-hour glucola. If you are given this test, you are asked to drink a very sweet orange drink, and one hour later a sample of your blood is drawn. If the blood sugar content is above a certain level, you might be at risk for gestational diabetes, and further tests are indicated.

Checking Blood Pressure and Performing the Urine Assay

At your weigh-in, you should expect to gain about one-half pound per week during the first 20 weeks of pregnancy and about a pound a week thereafter—approximately 30–35 pounds in total.

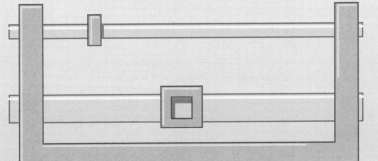

The urine sample that your practitioner requests at the beginning of every prenatal visit is tested with a *dipstick*. This is a thin cardboard stick that has been treated with a variety of chemicals that indicate the presence (or absence) of various substances. The medical assistant puts the dipstick into the urine and then evaluates the color changes the stick undergoes. The presence of either glucose or protein may indicate a need to do further blood tests.

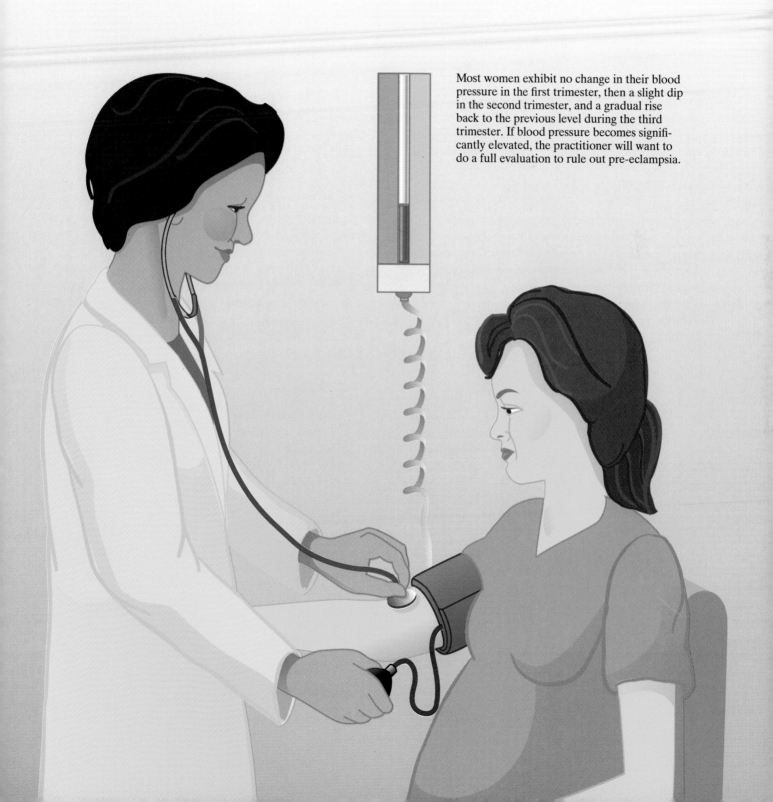

Most women exhibit no change in their blood pressure in the first trimester, then a slight dip in the second trimester, and a gradual rise back to the previous level during the third trimester. If blood pressure becomes significantly elevated, the practitioner will want to do a full evaluation to rule out pre-eclampsia.

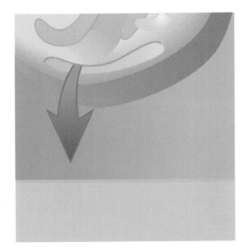

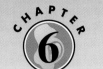

Screening for Fetal Abnormalities

THE ALPHAFETOPROTEIN (AFP) ASSAY is one of many screening tests that is used to detect fetal problems. AFP is a protein that the fetal liver produces. If there are any openings in the fetal skin, an unusually large amount of alphafetoprotein escapes into the amniotic fluid and crosses the placenta to the mother's blood stream.

The AFP assay measures the concentration of certain hormones in the mother's blood to predict whether the fetus is likely to have a neural tube defect or a chromosomal abnormality. *Neural tube defects* are the most common fetal abnormalities that result in high alphafetoprotein. These abnormalities arise when the neural tube, destined to become the spine, fails to close properly, and leaves an opening. If the opening is at the base of the spine, the defect is called *spina bifida*, which generally results in paralysis of the lower body. If the defect occurs at the upper end of the neural tube, brain abnormalities often associated with significant retardation can be expected.

Down's syndrome is an example of a chromosomal problem that results from an extra copy of chromosome 21. For reasons that are unclear, the babies of women who have abnormally low levels of AFP are more prone toward this condition than women with higher levels of AFP. Doctors made this unexpected finding when routine testing for neural tube defects was first instituted. After careful study, doctors concluded that AFP screening could be used routinely to detect Down's syndrome and other, similar chromosomal problems.

In the years since the test was introduced, several modifications have been made to it. To increase the test's accuracy, other hormones are also measured. In the AFP 2 test, human chorionic gonadotropin (HCG) is measured, and in the AFP 3 test, estriol is also measured. Both of these hormones are associated with the placenta. Fetuses afflicted with Down's syndrome tend to produce abnormal levels of these hormones as well as unusually low levels of alphafetoprotein.

It is important to remember that the AFP assay is a screening test, not a diagnosis. It can only predict the likelihood that a particular fetus has a neural tube defect or a chromosomal problem by comparing one test's results with thousands of other results. That's why the AFP assay does not report a diagnosis; it offers a probability.

The AFP Assay

It can be extremely frightening to be told that the AFP result is abnormal and that amniocentesis is recommended. But there is no need to panic when you keep this fact in mind: Abnormal test results suggest only a very small probability of Down's syndrome or neural tube defect. Most practitioners will recommend amniocentesis if the risk of Down's syndrome is higher than 1 in 270. Yet of all the amniocenteses done in that situation, only 1 out of 270 fetuses will actually be affected; that's much less than 1 percent.

Maternal age is an important factor in the probability calculation. The risk of Down's syndrome (*DS*) increases with increasing maternal age. Whatever the level of AFP, the older the mother, the higher the risk of Down's syndrome. For women over 35, the lab report will generally recommend amniocentesis regardless of AFP values.

EDC is the estimated date of confinement, or due date. *GA* is the gestational age. Several factors affect the interpretation of AFP results, including maternal weight, race, and whether or not the mother has diabetes. The number of fetuses also affects the amount of AFP expected. Twins are evaluated on a different probability scale, but it is not currently possible to interpret AFP results for triplets or more.

MS is maternal serum. *MOM* is multiple of the mean, a statistical term. Many laboratories will report the absolute values of the hormones that they measure. This test is clearly an AFP 2 test because it measured human chorionic gonadotropin (*HCG*) in addition to alphafetoprotein.

ONTD refers to open neural tube defect. This is the probability that this baby has an open neural tube defect such as spina bifida. This is an extremely small risk.

This is the most important part of the result. Notice that the result is expressed as a probability. This result means that this baby has a 1 in 1,200 chance of having Down's syndrome, which is a smaller probability than the baby of a 35-year old woman in her second trimester would have. If the probability is sufficiently high, your doctor or midwife will recommend ultrasound and amniocentesis tests to reach a diagnosis. The AFP assay cannot tell for certain whether a fetus is or is not affected.

Alphafetoprotein Assay

Age at EDC	26 years
GA on draw date	16.1 weeks
Race	Caucasian
MS-AFP	29.8 ng/ml
AFP MOM	0.56
HCG	19.70 mw/ml
HCG MOM	0.71
ONTD risk	<1:5,500
DS risk age only	1:600
DS risk all	1:1,200
DS interpret	

The risk for Down's syndrome based on age, AFP, and HCG is less than the second trimester risk of a woman at age 35.

An example of open neural tube defect

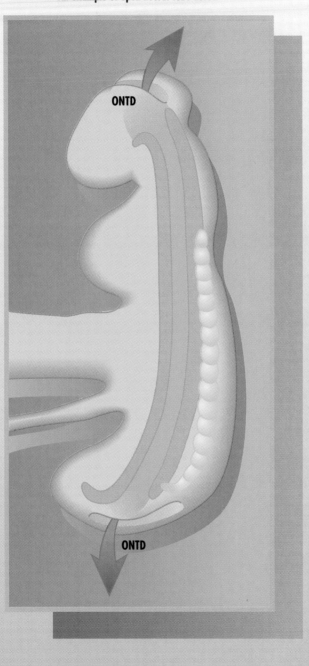

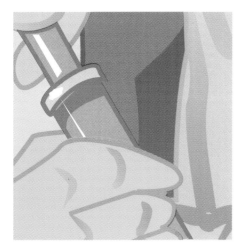

Amniocentesis

AMNIOCENTESIS IS THE name of the procedure in which a thin needle is inserted into the uterus to withdraw a small amount of amniotic fluid. The fetal skin cells found in the fluid are then analyzed for chromosomal abnormalities.

Most women who are recommended for an "amnio" fall into two large categories. Either they have received an abnormal result on the AFP screening test, or they are age 35 or older. Maternal age is an important risk factor for Down's syndrome; the incidence increases as maternal age increases. Furthermore, beginning with age 35, the risk of having a child with Down's syndrome exceeds the risk of injuring the pregnancy by the procedure. Under age 35, there is a greater risk of causing injury than there is of diagnosing a problem. Because of this risk, amniocentesis is not recommended for women under 35 unless the AFP result is abnormal.

It's hard not to be nervous about having an amnio, but it's actually a short and simple procedure. The entire process takes about 60 seconds. If you're like most people, your anxiety centers around the needle; many women are intimidated by its length. It's important to remember, though, that the amount of discomfort associated with a needle is related to the thickness of the needle, not the length. A very thin needle is used in amniocentesis; this minimizes possible injury to the fetus and decreases maternal discomfort.

Your doctor generally performs the amnio, and the procedure is always guided by ultrasound. This means the ultrasonographer monitors everything that happens, and guides your doctor in the placement of the needle. The risk of injury to the fetus is therefore very small.

Before beginning the amnio, the ultrasonographer does a complete evaluation of the fetus, just as if you were having a routine ultrasound. This time, though, he or she pays special attention to the fetus's location in the uterus. The ultrasonographer looks for a large "pocket" of fluid—a space where the needle can be inserted without coming close to the fetus. Some babies are more cooperative then others. Your baby might want to play tricks; every time a pocket is found, he or she might move into it, requiring a search for another pocket.

Once the pocket of fluid is identified, the ultrasonographer tells your doctor where the needle should be placed. Then, the overlying skin is "prepped" with betadine solution to minimize the risk of infection, and the doctor inserts a long, thin needle through the abdominal wall into the amniotic sac. He or she then withdraws a small amount of amniotic fluid and removes the needle. If you want to, you can watch the entire procedure.

The amniotic fluid that has been removed is sent to a special genetics laboratory. The fetal skin cells in the amniotic fluid, which have been shed during normal growth, are encouraged to grow and divide. Geneticists analyze the cells for the presence of chromosomal abnormalities. Growing the fetal cells and analyzing them can take anywhere from ten days to two weeks.

Amniocentesis

1 A very thin needle has been inserted through the uterine wall into the amniotic sac, and the fluid is being withdrawn. Inserting the needle takes only a few seconds. It takes approximately one minute to withdraw several teaspoons of fluid. The fluid is collected in a sterile syringe which is then capped, sealed, and taken to the genetics laboratory.

2 Notice how the needle has been inserted into a "pocket" of fluid. The fetus is far away from the needle, and there is very little risk of injury. The removal of a small amount of amniotic fluid has no impact on the baby. Since amniotic fluid is essentially fetal urine, it is constantly being "recycled." The fetus will replenish the fluid within 24 hours.

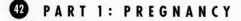

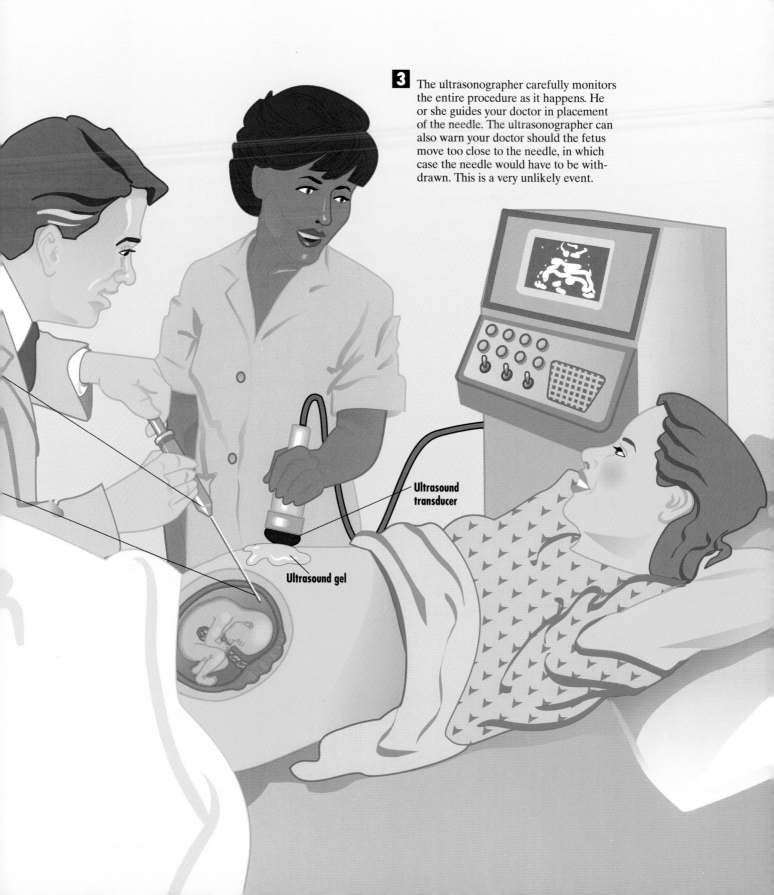

3 The ultrasonographer carefully monitors the entire procedure as it happens. He or she guides your doctor in placement of the needle. The ultrasonographer can also warn your doctor should the fetus move too close to the needle, in which case the needle would have to be withdrawn. This is a very unlikely event.

Ultrasound transducer

Ultrasound gel

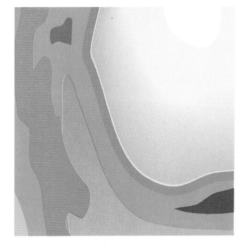

First-Trimester Bleeding

YOU'VE SHARED THE exciting news of your pregnancy with your friends and family. Then, one morning you wake up and notice a spot of blood on your underwear, and suddenly you're as frightened as you've ever been.

Don't panic. Although bleeding during pregnancy is never considered "normal," bleeding during the first trimester is very common. In fact, approximately one-quarter of all women who deliver healthy babies experience some bleeding in the first trimester.

Of course, bleeding can also be a sign of impending miscarriage, so it's important to discuss any bleeding with your midwife or doctor. She or he will probably wish to examine you (though not necessarily on an emergency basis), and will most likely order an ultrasound test to further evaluate your pregnancy.

What causes bleeding in the first trimester? And what type of bleeding is likely to indicate a miscarriage? One possible cause of light bleeding in the first trimester is related to the aggressive growth of the placenta. As the placenta establishes contact with the maternal circulation, some bleeding of the uterine wall may occur. This could cause retroplacental bleeding—a small collection of blood behind the placenta—and some of the blood may escape, causing vaginal bleeding.

There are several signs that may indicate the bleeding is a symptom of impending miscarriage. The most sensitive sign, and the one that your practitioner will probably ask you about first, is pain. In an impending miscarriage, bleeding is almost always associated with some lower abdominal cramping. Also, the volume of bleeding is generally quite a bit heavier in an impending miscarriage than in a normal pregnancy.

A blighted ovum is the most common cause of miscarriage. This term is somewhat misleading because it is not necessarily the ovum that is abnormal, but rather the combination of the ovum and sperm. The resulting chromosomal defect is so severe that although the pregnancy advances, development cannot proceed beyond the earliest stage. In most cases of blighted ovum, only the placental tissue, not the embryo, has developed. A blighted ovum does not indicate that either parent has a chromosomal abnormality. It affects only the fertilized ovum in question. There is no reason to believe that it will happen again in a future pregnancy.

This has important implications for dealing with miscarriage, both medically and psychologically. Because a blighted ovum is determined at the moment of conception, nothing can be done to prevent a miscarriage. If it's going to happen, it's going to happen. This also means that if you do have a miscarriage, you should never blame yourself. Virtually nothing you do can disrupt a normal pregnancy and, conversely, there is nothing you can do to save an abnormal one.

Lastly, bleeding may also be a sign of a much less common condition—ectopic pregnancy. *Ectopic pregnancy,* also known as *tubal pregnancy,* occurs when the fertilized ovum fails to travel all the way down the fallopian tube to the uterus. Instead, it implants in the wall of the fallopian tube. Such a pregnancy can never be successful. It may also cause serious health complications for the mother. An ultrasound test is often very helpful in diagnosing ectopic pregnancy.

Why Bleeding May Occur

Notice the small collection of fluid behind the placenta. This is blood that has welled up as the placenta continues to make contact with the maternal circulation. A little bit of blood may leak out from the collection: That's what causes the spotting that you see. The relatively small size of the collection is a good prognostic sign. Most of placenta is in contact with the uterine wall, providing oxygen and nutrients to the growing embryo.

When an ultrasound test is done to investigate first trimester bleeding, several important aspects of fetal growth are checked. The first check, to determine whether the embryonic heart can be seen beating, is the most important one, but the ultrasonographer also measures the embryo to determine if it is growing properly. The risk of miscarriage is much less if the heart can be seen beating and the embryo is growing properly.

The sac that holds the tiny embryo is smooth, round, and regular. This is another good sign. In an impending miscarriage, the embryonic sac is often distorted or crumpled.

If any blood escapes from behind the placenta and passes through the cervix, it will be detected by the mother as vaginal spotting.

A Blighted Ovum

Notice that the embryo is completely absent. There is probably a chromosomal defect so significant that no embryo ever developed, only placental tissue. This is the most important finding in a blighted ovum. The normal embryo would be clearly visible on ultrasound after five weeks gestation, although the heartbeat may not be seen until six weeks.

There is a large amount of blood behind the placenta. In fact, the placenta has almost totally detached from the uterine wall.

The embryonic sac is distorted, another sign that this pregnancy is about to miscarry.

Notice that the cervix is dilated and blood is freely passing through it. Once the cervix has dilated, a miscarriage is inevitable. In this case, no other outcome was possible—even before the cervix dilated. That's because there was never an embryo at all.

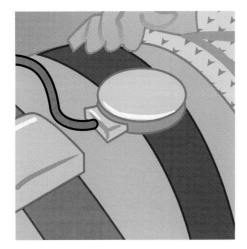

CHAPTER
9

Premature Labor

YOU'VE CIRCLED YOUR due date on the calendar and you're mentally counting down the weeks until the big day. Then something totally unexpected happens. Weeks before your due date you wake up in the middle of the night with contractions. You may be having premature labor.

Because no one yet understands the mechanism by which normal labor starts, we are often at a loss to explain why some women begin their labor before their due date. *Labor* is defined as regular uterine contractions which produce a change in the dilatation of the cervix. *Premature labor* is defined as labor that begins before 37 weeks of gestation.

Premature labor is often associated with other conditions. The most common, and easily treatable, is a urinary tract infection. Because the bladder is next to the uterus, an infection of the bladder can cause irritation of the uterus, leading to uterine contractions. Maternal dehydration is another, easily treatable cause of premature labor. Finally, the use of drugs, especially cocaine, may trigger premature labor.

What should you do if you think you might be starting labor prematurely? If you are experiencing repeated uterine contractions before 37 weeks of gestation, or if you are having menstrual-like cramping or constant low backache, you should contact your practitioner right away. To determine whether these are true premature contractions or just Braxton-Hicks contractions (the normal, painless contractions that occur in late pregnancy), she or he will ask you various questions—how often the contractions occur, how long they last, and how painful they are. In most cases, you will be asked to come to the office or the hospital for a complete evaluation.

The only way to accurately diagnose premature labor is by examining your cervix for any changes. Before the last month of pregnancy, the cervix is usually closed (although it may be slightly open in women who have previously given birth). The fetal monitor will be used both to check the fetal heart rate and to detect uterine contractions.

If there are any signs of premature labor, your physician will probably take several additional steps. Your urine will be checked for any sign of infection. You will be given fluid intravenously to counteract the effects of possible dehydration. Bed rest is a cornerstone of the treatment of premature labor. It is also easier to monitor the fetus and contractions while the expectant mother is in a bed. Amazingly enough, something as simple as this can be quite helpful. In most cases, no further evaluation or treatment is required. Most episodes of premature contractions (without any change in the cervix) will stop by themselves.

Occasionally, some women do experience true premature labor, which causes the cervix to open and puts the fetus at risk for premature delivery. If this occurs before 36 weeks of gestation, your practitioner will recommend treatment to prevent premature delivery. There are several different medications used for this purpose. The most common are ritodrine and terbutaline. They are initially given by injection, but if they succeed in stopping the contractions, they can be taken orally.

If there appears to be a risk of the fetus being delivered within a few days of the initial treatment, most obstetricians will also recommend the steroid betamethasone. The biggest hurdle facing premature newborns is whether their lungs are sufficiently mature to breathe on their own. Betamethasone speeds up the process of lung maturation, giving babies born early every possible advantage; however, it takes approximately 48 hours to act, so if it appears that delivery is imminent, betamethasone will not help.

Most cases of premature labor respond readily to treatment. Even if pregnancy can be prolonged only one additional week, it's often enough to give a premature newborn a big advantage. Special care nurseries can often support even the tiniest newborns (26 weeks gestation and sometimes younger) until they can breathe on their own.

Monitoring and Treating Premature Labor

3 The nurse is preparing to inject terbutaline subcutaneously—under the skin—of the mother's arm. A practitioner's evaluation has already determined that her cervix is dilated 1 cm. despite the fact that she is only 34 weeks pregnant. There is no evidence of a urinary tract infection, and the contractions have not stopped with hydration. Terbutaline is usually given in three injections, 20 minutes apart. In most cases, this is sufficient to stop the contractions. Then maintenance doses of terbutaline can be given orally every four hours.

1 cm.

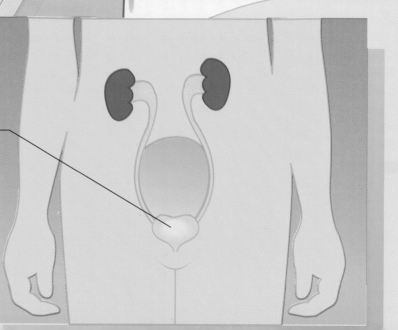

4 Notice how the bladder is immediately below the uterus. This explains why an infection in the bladder can irritate the uterus and cause premature contractions. The changes in surrounding structures caused by the growing uterus are probably responsible for the increased likelihood of infections of the entire urinary tract during pregnancy. Interestingly, pregnant women are much less likely to have symptoms from urinary tract infections (such as burning on urination) than nonpregnant women.

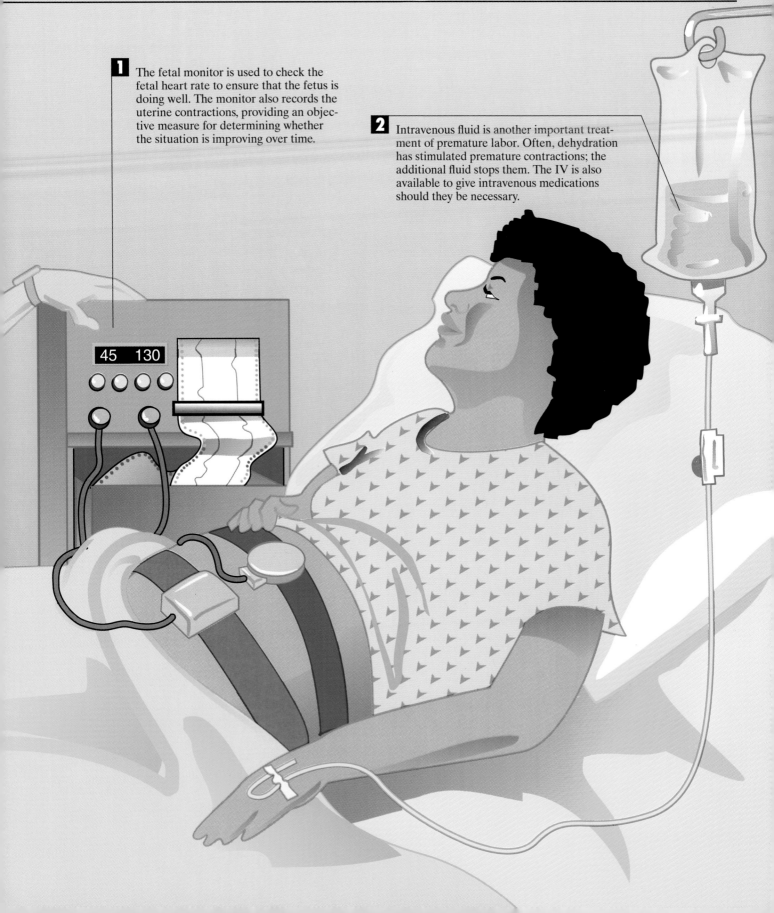

1 The fetal monitor is used to check the fetal heart rate to ensure that the fetus is doing well. The monitor also records the uterine contractions, providing an objective measure for determining whether the situation is improving over time.

2 Intravenous fluid is another important treatment of premature labor. Often, dehydration has stimulated premature contractions; the additional fluid stops them. The IV is also available to give intravenous medications should they be necessary.

45   130

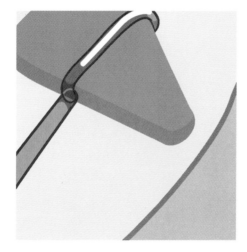

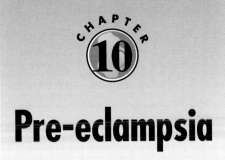

Pre-eclampsia

E VERY VISIT TO your doctor or midwife starts with the same routine, a blood pressure check, weight check, and the testing of a urine sample. These simple tests are designed to detect pre-eclampsia.

Pre-eclampsia (also known as toxemia or pregnancy-induced hypertension) is a disease that affects only pregnant women. This disease is much more common in first pregnancies, and is more likely to affect women at either end of their reproductive years—that is, both very young and older first-time mothers. Pre-eclampsia was originally characterized by elevated blood pressure, edema (swelling), and protein in the urine. As our understanding of this condition has grown, additional signs and symptoms have been identified. The most important of these is extreme sensitivity of the nervous system, which may cause seizures. Pre-eclampsia can also cause abnormalities in blood clotting and liver function.

Blood pressure measurement is expressed with two values, one value "over" another value. The upper number is the systolic pressure, and the lower number is the diastolic pressure. A typical blood pressure for a pregnant woman might be 110/70, or 110 "over" 70. If the diastolic pressure (bottom number) rises into the 90s and is sustained at that level, the possibility of pre-eclampsia must be considered. A sustained diastolic pressure above 100 is usually indicative of a severe case of pre-eclampsia.

It is important to remember, however, that a diagnosis of pre-eclampsia can only be made by comparing changes in a pregnant woman's blood pressure with her own blood pressure earlier in the pregnancy (preferably the first trimester). What is normal for one woman may be abnormal for another.

In the days before pre-eclampsia could be treated, serious complications often developed. These included seizures, strokes, and kidney damage. Today, these complications are almost never seen. Pre-eclampsia is usually diagnosed early and treated effectively. For example, women who have moderate to severe symptoms may be treated with magnesium sulfate administered through an intravenous line; this treatment will usually prevent seizures.

If your doctor or midwife has any reason to believe that you might be developing pre-eclampsia, you will get a thorough physical exam and a variety of blood tests that can give you more information about the course of the disease. You will also be advised about certain symptoms to watch for, including headache, blurry vision, and upper abdominal pain. These symptoms may indicate that your blood pressure is too high. If necessary, your practitioner may prescribe drugs, such as hydralazine, to lower your blood pressure.

Your practitioner will also recommend bed rest on your left side. In mild cases of pre-eclampsia, bed rest may be all that is needed to lower your blood pressure until delivery. The reason the left side is preferred is that this position takes the weight of the uterus off the major blood vessels which lie behind it, allowing maximum blood flow to the uterus and placenta.

No one knows what causes pre-eclampsia or why some women are more likely to get it than others. Many doctors believe that pre-eclampsia is an abnormal maternal reaction to placental tissue. It is most common in first time mothers, particularly those at either end of the reproductive years, teenagers and women over 35. It is well-known that pre-eclampsia is rapidly cured (within 24–48 hours) by the delivery of the baby and placenta.

If your blood pressure is very high, or if it continues to rise despite bed rest, you may be admitted to the hospital. There, a decision will be made about whether or not your baby should be delivered early. Many factors go into making the decision, including how far you are from your due date, whether your baby is being adversely affected by your high blood pressure, and, most importantly, how the disease is affecting you. Anyone who has significant symptoms or very abnormal blood test results will probably have labor induced. That's because the disease will only get worse until after the baby has been delivered.

Labor is usually induced intravenously with pitocin. *Pitocin* is a synthetic hormone that is chemicaly identical to the hormone *oxytocin*, which causes contractions. Women who have pre-eclampsia tend to have a more rapid response to Pitocin, and possibly, a faster labor; it's almost as if the uterus senses the need for an early delivery. If labor cannot be induced successfully, or if further problems develop during labor, a Caesarean section may be necessary.

Symptoms of Pre-eclampsia

The most important symptom of pre-eclampsia is extreme sensitivity of the nervous system. This may even cause seizures. The woman in this picture had a blood pressure of approximately 110/70 during the first 36 weeks of pregnancy. When she visited her practitioner, her blood pressure was 140/90. This immediately raised the concerns about pre-eclampsia. However, elevated blood pressure alone, unless it is very high, is not enough to reach a diagnosis. The practitioner will undertake a search for other signs and symptoms before reaching a conclusion.

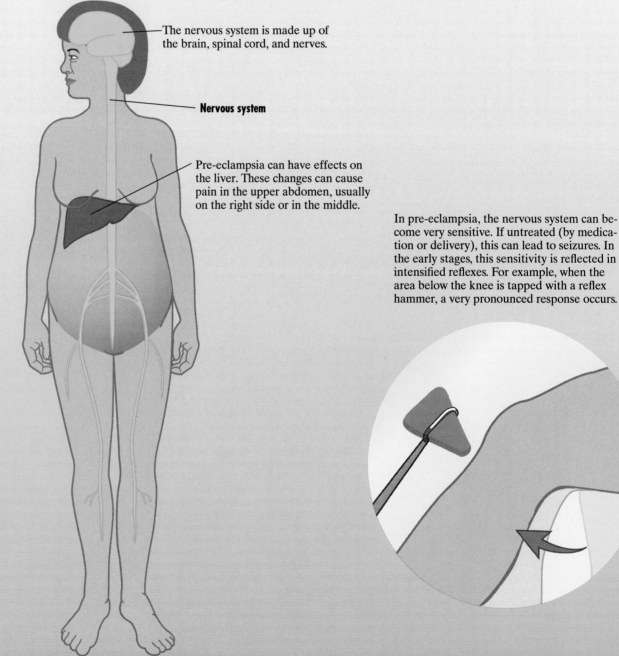

The nervous system is made up of the brain, spinal cord, and nerves.

Nervous system

Pre-eclampsia can have effects on the liver. These changes can cause pain in the upper abdomen, usually on the right side or in the middle.

In pre-eclampsia, the nervous system can become very sensitive. If untreated (by medication or delivery), this can lead to seizures. In the early stages, this sensitivity is reflected in intensified reflexes. For example, when the area below the knee is tapped with a reflex hammer, a very pronounced response occurs.

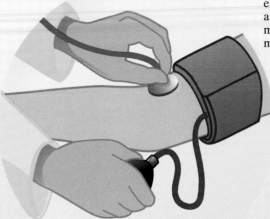

The most critical symptom of pre-eclampsia is elevated blood pressure. No one can actually *feel* a rise in blood pressure, but high blood pressure may cause several warning signs. The most common signs are headache and blurry vision.

One of the most important signs of pre-eclampsia is edema or swelling. Many pregnant women's feet swell, especially at the end of the day, but swelling without other signs or symptoms is not a cause for concern. In pre-eclampsia, however, the swelling is usually more pronounced and often affects the hands and the face. It is always accompanied by other symptoms, most often by elevated blood pressure.

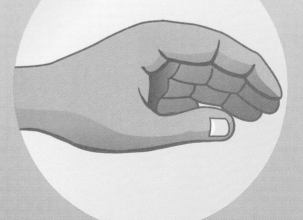

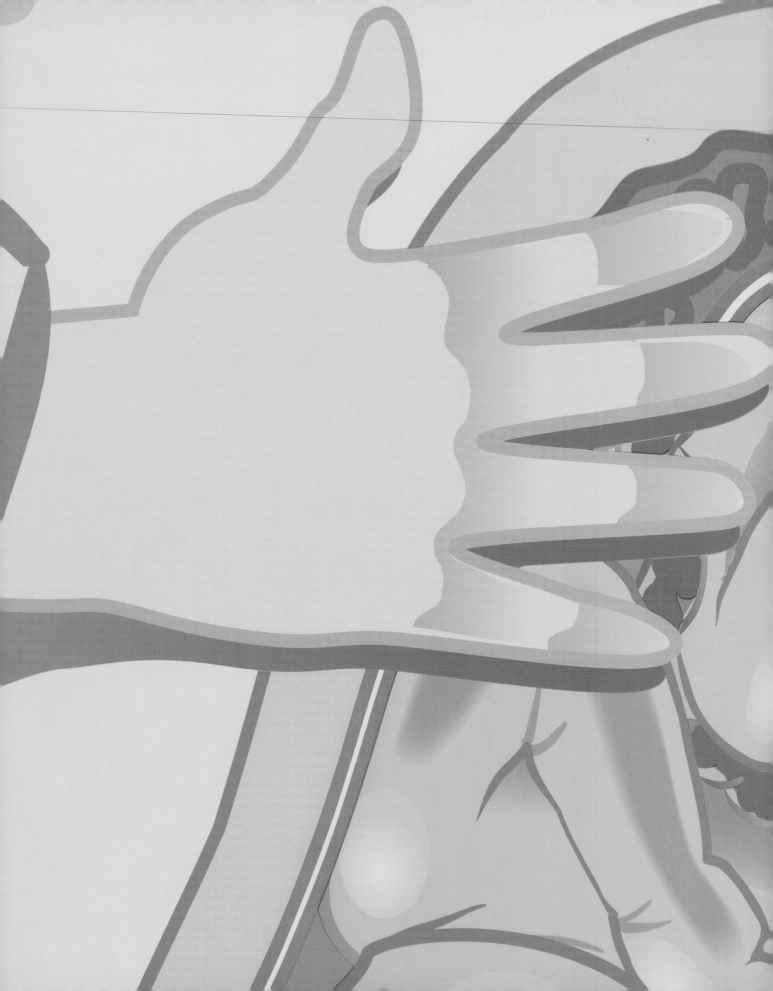

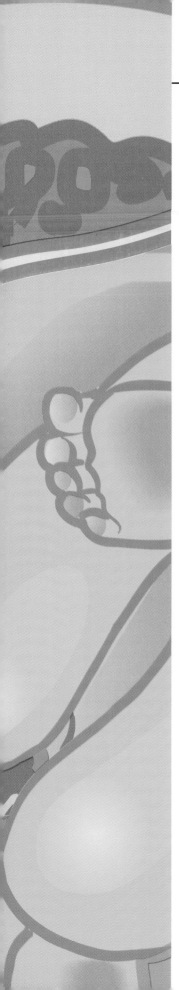

LABOR AND DELIVERY

2

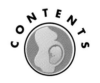

CONTENTS

THE WEEKS AND months have passed, and your due date is rapidly approaching. The event that you have waited, planned, and hoped for is almost here. It seems that everywhere you go people have stories to share about their own birth experiences. Some sound sublime and others sound, well, just awful. Why do some women have such great labors and others such miserable ones? What can you do to ensure the best possible labor and delivery?

Someone once described labor as dependent on the three Ps—pelvis, passenger, and power—and that's not far from the truth. These three factors, individually and in combination, determine the length of your labor and whether you ultimately might need a Caesarean section.

The first P stands for the pelvis. What is meant here is the bony pelvis, the bone structure that supports the lower body and through which the baby's head must pass during labor. The mother's soft tissues will stretch during labor and delivery, but the pelvic opening, being bone, will not. Not surprisingly, women with a small pelvic opening will find it difficult, if not impossible, to deliver a large baby.

Of course, most women have a pelvic opening that is more than adequate to deliver an average baby. Your doctor or midwife will most likely do an internal exam a few weeks before your delivery date to assess your pelvis. The important thing is not the absolute size of the pelvic opening, but rather its relative size compared to the size of the baby's head.

The second P refers to the passenger (your baby). While it will be more difficult to deliver a larger baby than a smaller one, it's not the baby's weight that counts, it's the size and the position of the fetal head that are most important. Obviously, a bigger fetus will have a bigger head, but there are ways for the fetus to position his or her head that will make it easier to pass through the pelvis.

During the course of labor, while the cervix is dilating, the pressure of the uterine contractions encourages the fetus to assume the position in which the smallest possible diameter of the head is "presenting," or coming first. Not all babies cooperate, however, and if yours decides to go through the pelvis facing up or turned sideways rather than down toward your back, your labor will be longer and more difficult. It is much easier to deliver a baby whose head is tucked down on his or her chest rather than one attempting to come out face first (fortunately, this is a very uncommon position).

Even if the fetal head is large (compared to the mother's pelvis), or is in a less than ideal position, all is not lost. That's because the fetal head is capable of changing shape during labor. The bones of the fetal skull are not fastened to each other the way they are in the adult skull. The bones are free to move in relation to each other, allowing the fetal head to conform to the size and shape of the pelvic opening. This process is known as *molding*. Molding takes time, which is why a baby born after a long labor has a "cone-head." The head actually gets longer and thinner to fit through the pelvic opening! It will return to normal shape in 24–48 hours, without any harm to the baby.

The final P stands for power—that is, the power of the uterine contractions. Not all contractions are alike; some are stronger than others. Usually, as labor progresses, the contractions become longer and stronger. However, some women never have strong enough contractions to get the job done, that is, to cause the cervix to dilate the necessary 10 cm. and to push the baby out. If your practitioner suspects that your contractions are not strong enough, she or he can strengthen them by giving you Pitocin, a synthetic version of the hormone oxytocin, which causes contractions.

If you need Pitocin, you will probably realize it at the same time that your practitioner does. Perhaps you've been in labor for many hours without dilation of your cervix, or maybe you made great progress until a certain point but then, despite additional hours of labor, nothing changes. Pitocin may then get you back on track by causing the contractions to become stronger and more effective.

However, there's no guarantee that Pitocin will cause continued progress. The uterus is an amazing organ, and it appears to be able to sense if the fetus is too large to deliver. In such cases, the cervix will not dilate any further, even with Pitocin. Then, it is clear that a C-section needs to be done.

What can you do to improve the course of your labor? Well, not much. The size of your pelvis was determined long ago, and you don't have any control over the size of the baby or the position it decides to assume. There are, however, a number of things you can do to ensure that your contractions are as strong and effective as they can be. The following seven chapters discuss the process of labor and delivery in detail, from the first contraction to delivery of the placenta, placing special emphasis on the things that you can do to encourage a smooth and efficient labor.

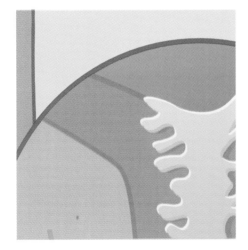

CHAPTER 11

Before Labor Begins

HAS THE BABY dropped yet? Friends and complete strangers are asking the same question. What are they talking about? How will you know the answer to this question?

As the end of pregnancy draws near, the fetus is likely to take a position that will be favorable for the coming journey. Over 95 percent of all fetuses will be facing head down, with their chins tucked on their chests. Some babies, particularly those of first-time mothers, will literally drop into the pelvic opening. The cervix may not have dilated, and the fetus is still totally within the uterus, but the fetal head is now nestled *within* the pelvic opening instead of above it. Doctors and midwives refer to this process as *engagement.*

Engagement is also known as *lightening,* probably because it provides relief from some common pregnancy symptoms. When your baby drops, pressure on your stomach and diaphragm drops, too. You will probably have less heartburn and shortness of breath. Of course, these symptoms may merely be exchanged for new ones. You may feel increased pelvic pressure, and some women complain that it's hard to walk because it feels like the baby's head is between their legs. However, it's important to remember that many women have no change in their symptoms and never even notice when the fetal head engages. In any event, it is quite possible that the baby will not drop until labor begins.

There are other signs that the time for labor may be drawing near. For example, the *mucous plug,* which has kept the inside of the uterus sealed off from the vagina, falls out as the cervix begins to soften and thin in preparation for labor. The mucous plug may fall out hours or even days before labor begins. Sometimes the membranes of the amniotic sac rupture (this is called "breaking your water") minutes or hours before labor begins. If your membranes rupture, you should call your practitioner. Some doctors and midwives prefer that you come in for examination right away. Others will advise you to wait at home to see if labor begins spontaneously.

Some women exhibit other physical symptoms that signal labor is approaching, including diarrhea, low-back ache, or abdominal cramping. There are many who believe that impending labor causes psychological changes as well. Some women are seized with the nesting instinct in the hours and days before labor begins: They are suddenly consumed with the urge to clean and arrange things, when just a few days before they were too exhausted to move.

Can you do anything deliberately to start your own labor? Well, there are a lot of old (and new) wives' tales that you can consider. Some women insist that spicy food started their labors, and others claim it was because they dosed themselves with castor oil. Then there are those who swear by sex, reasoning that even if it doesn't work, at least they'll have a good time. Unfortunately, it's not likely that any of these home remedies are effective. Labor starts when the baby is ready—and not one second before.

Fetus with Unengaged Head

Labor has not begun yet, nor has the cervix dilated, in either of the pictures shown here.

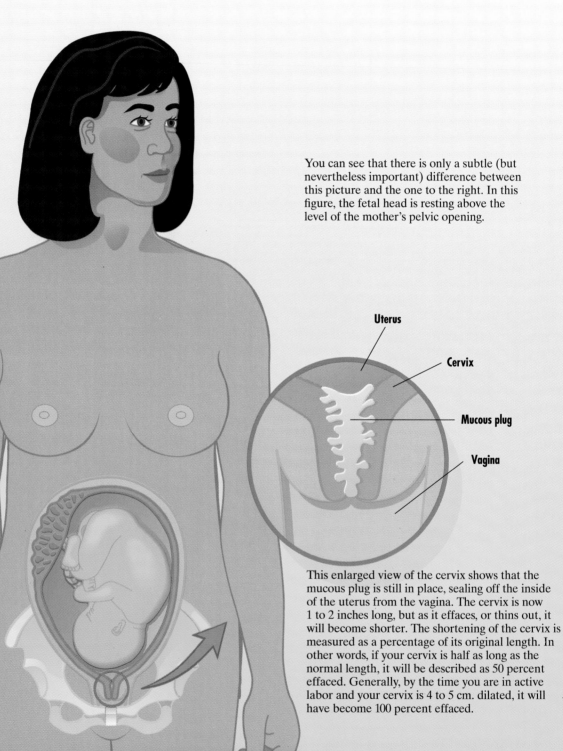

You can see that there is only a subtle (but nevertheless important) difference between this picture and the one to the right. In this figure, the fetal head is resting above the level of the mother's pelvic opening.

Uterus

Cervix

Mucous plug

Vagina

This enlarged view of the cervix shows that the mucous plug is still in place, sealing off the inside of the uterus from the vagina. The cervix is now 1 to 2 inches long, but as it effaces, or thins out, it will become shorter. The shortening of the cervix is measured as a percentage of its original length. In other words, if your cervix is half as long as the normal length, it will be described as 50 percent effaced. Generally, by the time you are in active labor and your cervix is 4 to 5 cm. dilated, it will have become 100 percent effaced.

Fetus with Engaged Head

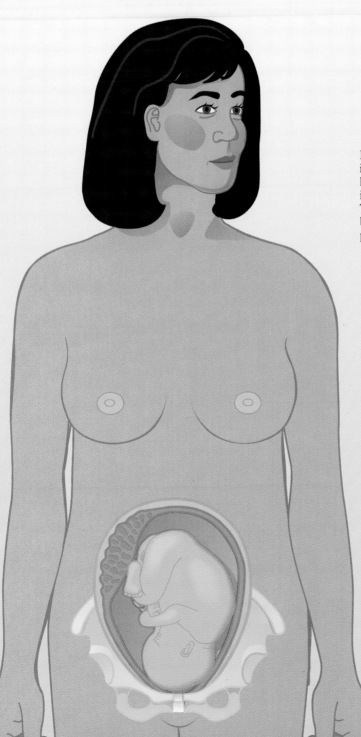

In this figure, the fetal head has dropped into the pelvic opening. As the baby drops lower in the pelvis, pressure on the abdominal organs and the diaphragm decreases. The mother may feel less shortness of breath and heartburn. The pressure on the pelvic organs, though, may be increased.

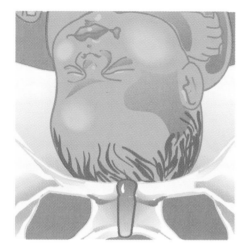

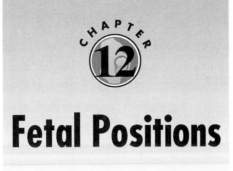

Fetal Positions

FETAL POSITION PLAYS a very important role in determining the course of labor, and in whether the fetus will ultimately fit through the mother's pelvic opening. When we consider the best position of the fetus for delivery, we begin to understand why some positions make vaginal delivery more difficult, some make it more dangerous, and why some positions are completely undeliverable.

During normal vaginal delivery, there is a relatively tight fit between the largest part of the baby, almost always its head, and the mother's pelvic opening. If the baby can position his or her head in such a way as to present the smallest possible diameter, labor will progress more smoothly.

Neither the fetal nor the infant head is perfectly round. When you dress a baby, you take this into account without even thinking about it. It is much easier to pull on those cute little T-shirts starting at the back of the baby's head, because the head is naturally egg shaped. Starting over the "point" at the back of the head makes it easier to slip clothes on.

In exactly the same way, starting labor with the "point" at the back of the baby's head leading the way makes it easier for the head to slip through the pelvic opening. In the ideal position for labor, the fetus is head down, facing the mother's back, with its chin tucked on its chest. This position is known as *occiput anterior*, which signifies that the occiput (back) of the fetal skull rests against the anterior (front) portion of the mother's pelvis.

Of course, lots of babies don't cooperate. Their chins may not be tucked, a position known as *deflexed head*, or their heads may be turned to one side or another in the *occiput transverse* position. Some may face away from their mothers' backs in the *occiput posterior* position. In all these cases, labor is likely to be slower and more difficult, because the position of the baby's head creates a slightly larger diameter that must pass through the pelvic opening. When the fetus is in the occiput posterior position, the mother is likely to experience back labor, feeling the contractions more in her back than in the front of her body.

Then, there are some babies who are totally uncooperative. They choose to assume the breech position (this position is also referred to as a *breech presentation*). This means that the baby's bottom, not the head, comes first, which makes for a more difficult delivery than those in which the baby assumes one of the other possible positions.

It's easy to understand why the breech presentation is potentially dangerous. On the one hand, the breech (the baby's rear end) may easily pass through the pelvic opening because of its smaller diameter. However, the head, which is always larger, may then get trapped in the pelvic opening, which constitutes an obstetric emergency.

A baby cannot breathe until the head is successfully delivered. Therefore, strenuous efforts must be made to deliver the head as quickly as possible in a breech presentation. Unfortunately, these same efforts, which are required to save the baby's life, may cause serious, permanent injury. This is the main reason that breech vaginal deliveries are considered hazardous. For more detail on breech presentations, see Chapter 26.

It's interesting to note that a baby that can only be delivered with great difficulty from the breech position would fit easily through the pelvic opening, if it arrived head first. This is true because the head would have had an opportunity to mold itself to the pelvic opening during the long hours of labor. This same head has had no time to mold if the breech has been delivered first. Furthermore, the umbilical cord is compressed between the baby's body and the walls of the vagina, depriving the baby of oxygen.

Finally, there are some positions that are just undeliverable, no matter how long or strong the contractions are. A transverse lie is such a position. The fetal back may be pressing against the cervix, or perhaps a shoulder is coming through first. Clearly, the entire baby will never fit through the pelvic opening back first. If the baby cannot be coaxed into assuming a more favorable position, a C-section is the only choice.

There is no reason to worry if your baby's head is not down before 36 weeks of gestation. Before then, there is a lot of room for the baby to turn around, and it will most likely do just that. However, if your practitioner finds the baby to be in the breech or transverse position in the last few weeks of pregnancy, he or she can try to manually turn the baby to the head-down position. This procedure is called *version* and it is successful more than 50 percent of the time. Version will be considered in detail in Chapter 26.

Remember, fetal position is just one of many factors that determine the course and outcome of labor. Because parents and practitioners have little or no control over these factors, everyone involved must be flexible. In labor, the baby runs the show. Parents and care givers can only respond to its demands.

Fetal Positions

Vertex, left occiput anterior   This is the most common fetal position at the beginning of labor. Vertex is the technical term for the head-first position. Left occiput anterior means that the occiput (back) of the fetal skull rests against the left anterior (front) portion of the mother's pelvis. This position is the most favorable for a vaginal delivery. No one understands how the fetus naturally assumes the most favorable position, but there are those who believe that this position is the most comfortable for the fetus even before labor begins.

Vertex, occiput posterior   Notice that the fetus is facing away from the mother instead of toward her. This position is slightly more difficult for vaginal delivery. Also, back labor is much more likely when the fetus is in the occiput posterior position. In back labor, the mother feels most of the pain of the contractions in her back, not in her abdomen.

Frank breech   This is the most common breech presentation, and the one that is most favorable for vaginal delivery. In this position, the bottom comes first and the legs are folded up onto the baby's abdomen. Babies delivered from this position, either by vaginal delivery or by Caesarean section, may have legs that stick straight up in the air for the first few hours after birth.

Transverse lie   This particular fetus is in the transverse position with its back facing down. You can see that it is impossible for the fetus to fit through the pelvis back first. A vaginal delivery cannot take place from this position. The fetus must either be turned to the vertex position (preferably) or to the frank breech position, or be delivered by Caesarean section.

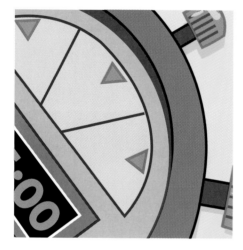

CHAPTER 13

What Happens in Early Labor

STARTING LABOR IS a little like starting your car on a cold January morning; sometimes it takes a few tries before it "turns over." A few women start true labor abruptly, but many experience one or two episodes of false labor before the real thing begins. Since that's the case, you might worry about whether you are really in labor. There is no reason to worry, though, because nobody ever missed her own labor. If you are not sure you're in labor, you probably aren't. And even if you are, you'll most likely have plenty of time to get to the hospital.

How can you tell the difference between false labor and true labor? In true labor, you will feel regular uterine contractions, every 5 minutes or even more frequently. Each contraction will last at least 45 seconds. These regular contractions must continue for at least an hour before you should consider it to be labor; even then, you may be wrong. In true labor, the contractions become increasingly long, stronger, and more frequent. In response to these contractions, the cervix thins out and begins to dilate (open).

Many women who have already delivered one baby find that their next labor is considerably shorter; it's like getting extra credit for having been through it once before. These women are advised to call their doctor when they have had regular contractions for an hour—even if the contractions are further apart than every five minutes.

The average first labor lasts for 12–18 hours before the cervix dilates to 10 cm., and it usually takes an additional 1–2 hours to push the baby out. Therefore, not much is likely to happen in the first hour. In false labor, the contractions weaken or occur less frequently. In this case, the contractions will eventually stop, only to start again hours (or even days) later.

Progress is usually very slow during the early phase of labor, which is also called the *latent phase*. Many contractions and a lot of time are required to make the cervix dilate the first few centimeters. However, each subsequent centimeter of dilatation takes less time to occur than the previous dilations. Stronger contractions facilitate increased dilation as they intensify during the course of labor.

You probably will be relatively comfortable during the early part of the latent phase of labor. Walking around is strongly encouraged, because it naturally stimulates labor. As the hours pass, though, you may become frustrated by the slow progress and the increasing discomfort. You may become so tired and fed up to the point where that pain medication seems very appealing. Unfortunately, pain medication or an epidural given in the latent phase is likely to slow down your labor, possibly so much so that medical intervention (such as administering Pitocin to induce labor) may be required to get it back on track again. (For more on epidural anesthesia, see Chapter 24.) This is why it's important to try to hang on until the active phase of labor begins. At that point, pain medication or an epidural cannot slow down or stop your labor.

The Latent Phase of Labor

The woman shown here has been in labor for several hours. She stayed at home for the first three hours, until the contractions became 5 minutes apart. Her practitioner examined her when she first came to the hospital and found her to be 2 cm. dilated. Because she is still in the early part of the latent phase, she was encouraged to walk around to stimulate labor naturally.

When the mother was admitted to the hospital, the fetus was assessed using the electronic fetal monitor. This is a standard practice that will be discussed in detail in Chapter 18. The fetus has been tolerating the relatively mild contractions of early labor without any difficulty so there's no reason to monitor the fetus continuously at this point in labor.

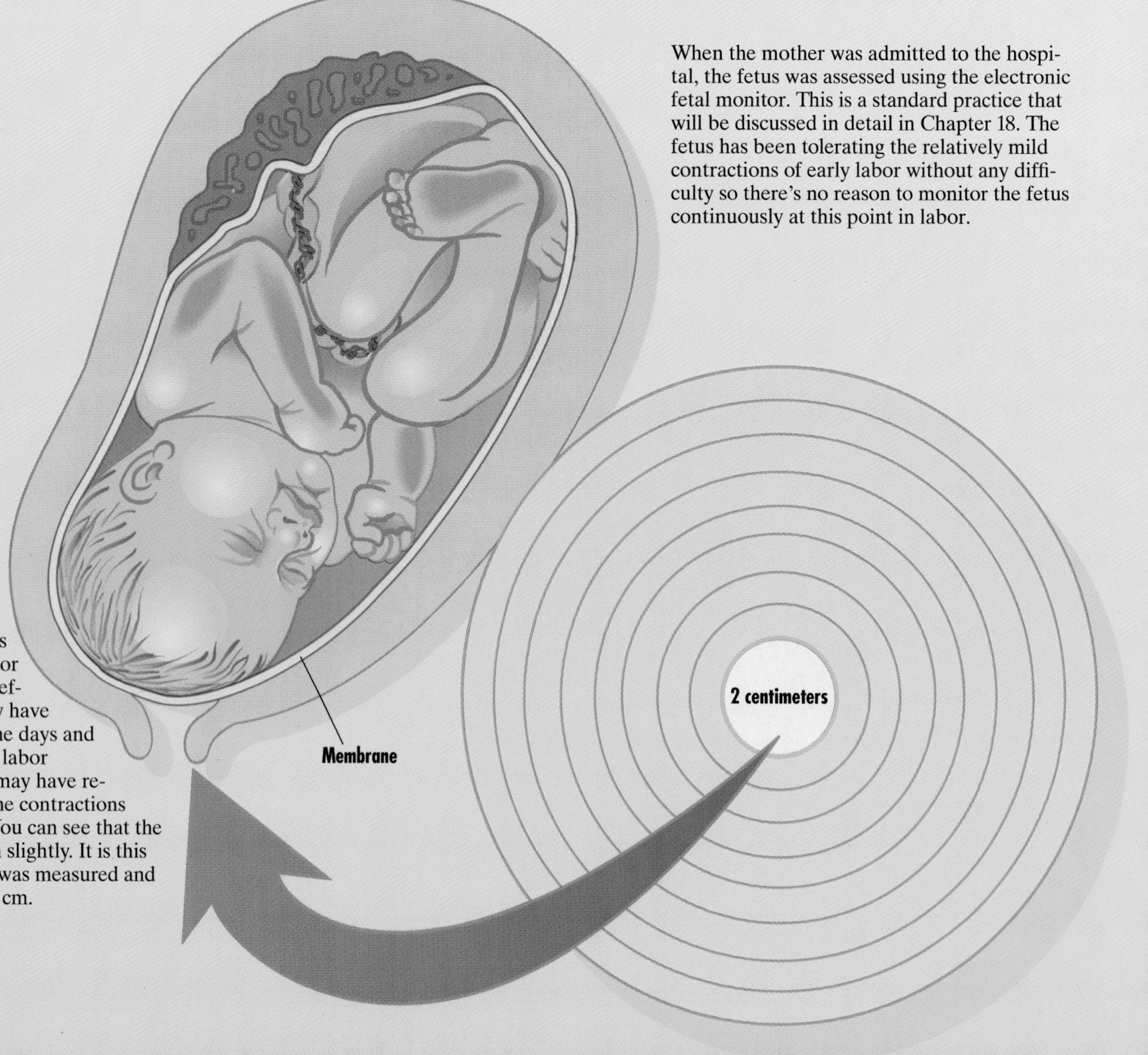

The cervix has become thin, or effaced. This effacement may have occurred in the days and weeks before labor started, or it may have resulted from the contractions themselves. You can see that the cervix is open slightly. It is this opening that was measured and found to be 2 cm.

Membrane

2 centimeters

The father can be a very supportive presence. Not only are his excitement and involvement reassuring to the mother, there are also lots of practical things he can do. For example, many expectant women find back massage very helpful in easing the discomforts of labor.

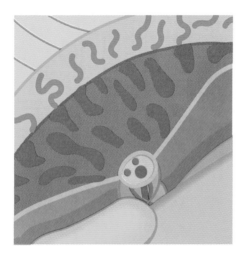

How the Uterus Contracts

YOU RECOGNIZE CONTRACTIONS when you feel them because the pain and pressure are unmistakable. But what are contractions? How do they cause the cervix to dilate? What happens to the fetus during a contraction?

In order to understand contractions, it is important to consider how the uterus acts on the fetus. Think of the uterus as a muscular bag that is made up of involuntary muscle. You cannot flex or release this type of muscle as you can the muscles that control the movements of your limbs. Therefore, you can't strengthen these involuntary muscles by exercising before labor. If the hormone oxytocin is present in sufficient quantities, it will cause the involuntary muscle of the uterus to contract in a regular pattern.

The involuntary muscle of the uterus is divided into two parts. The upper part is the *active segment;* it contracts and pushes against the baby. The lower part of this muscular bag is known as the *passive segment.* This part actually remains relaxed during the contraction. The net effect is to push the fetal head against the cervix. Repeated pressure of the fetal head on the cervix causes the cervix to thin out (efface) and then retract around the fetal head. The fetus is not so much forced out of the bag, as the bag pulls up around its head.

The average diameter of a fetal head is 10 cm. That's why the cervix is not considered to be fully dilated until 10 cm. is reached. At that point, the cervix has thinned out so much that there is no cervix left to hold back the fetal head, and the baby can be pushed out. If you start pushing before 10 cm. dilation is reached, you may damage the cervix.

When the involuntary muscle of the active segment contracts, it also compresses the blood vessels that travel through the uterine wall and carry oxygen to the placenta. This means that during the contraction, no oxygen can be transferred to the fetus. It's as if the fetus holds its breath for the length of the contraction. However, the placenta is designed to compensate for this under normal circumstances. Enough oxygen is transported to the fetus *between* contractions to allow the fetus to tolerate each contraction without any difficulty.

If there is a problem with the placenta—perhaps the baby is overdue and the placenta is a bit "worn out"—the fetus may not tolerate the contractions nearly so well. In such a case, the fetus may receive the minimally acceptable amount of oxygen between contractions, but may have no reserves with which to "hold its breath" during contractions. In this case, the baby's heart rate may drop immediately after each contraction. Continuous fetal heart rate monitoring can alert your practitioner to this potentially dangerous situation. Often, administering supplemental oxygen to the mother will correct the problem.

If this problem persists despite additional oxygen, the doctor or midwife must consider the possibility that the fetus will remain oxygen-deprived for the rest of labor. This condition is known as *fetal distress*. If there are many hours of labor remaining (perhaps the mother's cervix is dilated to only 5 cm.), a C-section would most likely be indicated to prevent the possibility of brain damage caused by chronic oxygen deprivation.

How the Uterus Contracts

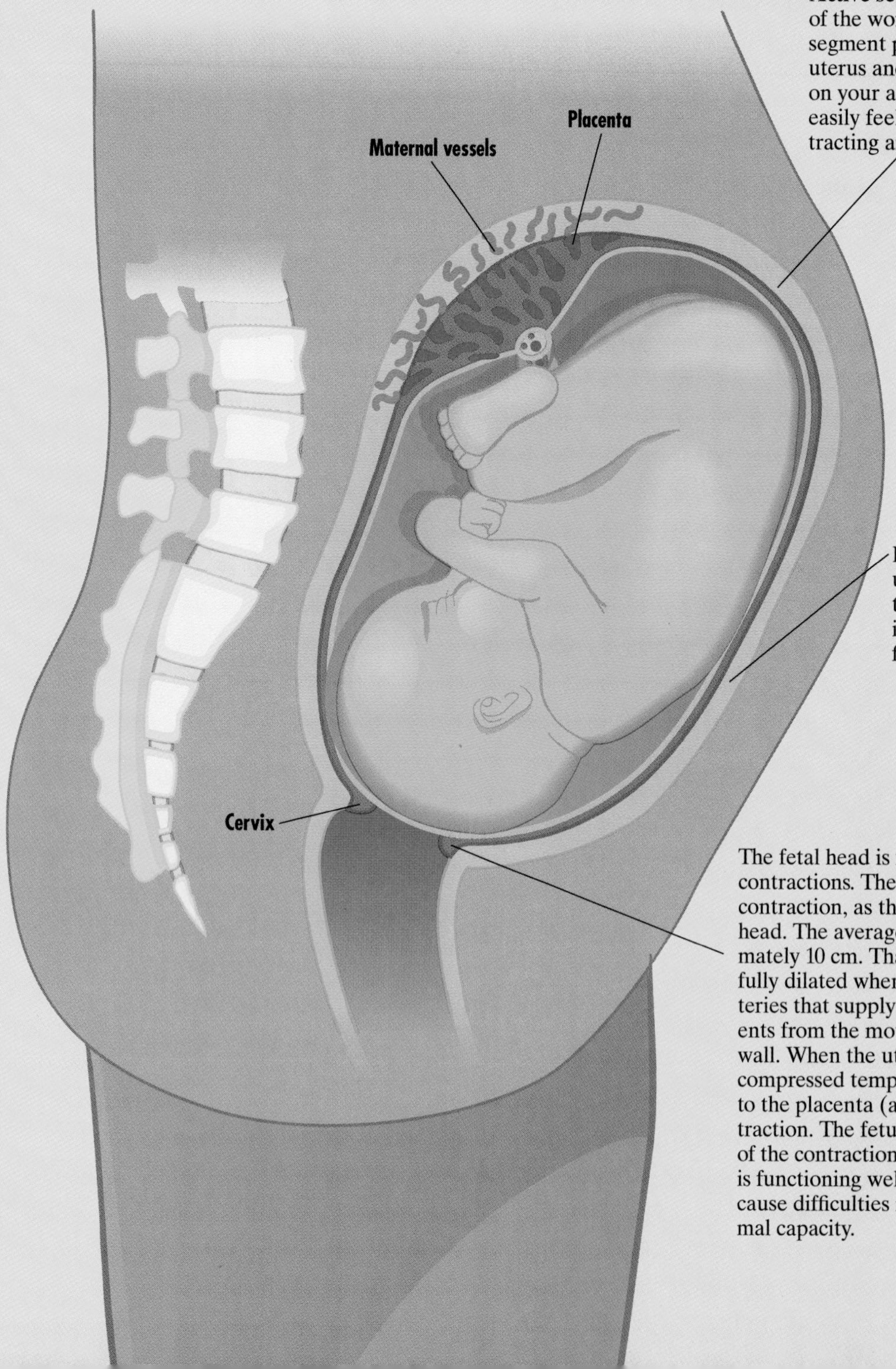

Active segment This part of the uterus does most of the work when the uterus contracts. The active segment pushes the fetus into the lower part of the uterus and against the cervix. If you put your hand on your abdomen during a contraction, you will easily feel the muscle of the active segment contracting and pushing on the fetus.

Placenta

Maternal vessels

Passive segment This part of the uterus does not exert much force on the fetus during a contraction. Because it is relatively relaxed, it allows the fetus to descend against the cervix.

Cervix

The fetal head is forced against the cervix during the contractions. The cervix dilates a bit more with each contraction, as the uterus pulls up around the fetal head. The average diameter of the fetal head is approximately 10 cm. That's why the cervix is considered to be fully dilated when 10 cm. is reached. Notice how the arteries that supply the placenta with oxygen and nutrients from the mother's bloodstream traverse the uterine wall. When the uterus contracts, these blood vessels are compressed temporarily. Oxygen cannot be transported to the placenta (and thereby to the fetus) during a contraction. The fetus must "hold its breath" for the length of the contraction. This poses no problem if the placenta is functioning well between contractions, but it can cause difficulties if the placenta is not working at optimal capacity.

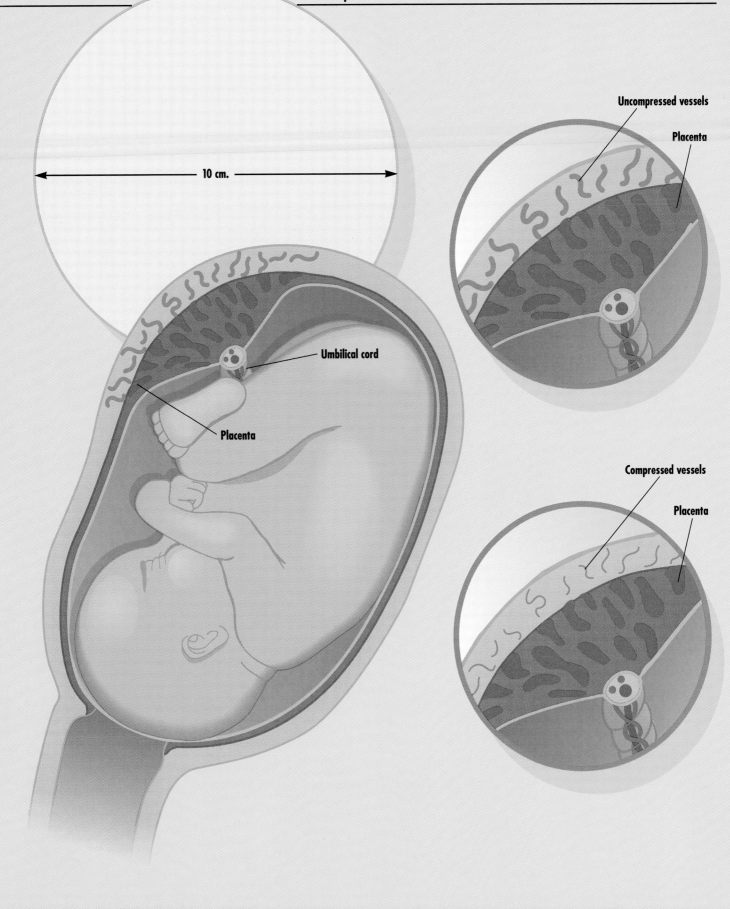

10 cm.

Umbilical cord

Placenta

Uncompressed vessels

Placenta

Compressed vessels

Placenta

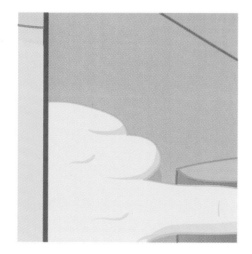

How Your Practitioner Checks Your Cervix

YOU'VE BEEN IN labor for several hours and you are anxious to find out about your progress. You might get very excited when your practitioner agrees that it's time to check your cervix. You watch him or her don the sterile glove, you feel fingers being inserted into your vagina, and you hear the approving announcement that you have dilated to 4 cm. But what on earth did the practitioner just do? What does the number mean?

When doctors or midwives do vaginal exams, they are able to feel three different things with their fingers. They measure *cervical dilation*, which is the amount that the cervix has opened, and *fetal station*, which is the relationship between the largest part of the fetal head and the midpoint of the maternal pelvis. If the cervix is dilated far enough, they can even feel the position of the fetal head. (See Chapter 12 for details on fetal positions.)

Cervical dilation is easy to measure. After identifying the cervical opening overlaying the fetal head, the practitioner slips one or two fingers into the opening cervix. If only one finger can be admitted, the cervix is approximately 1 cm. dilated. If two fingers can be placed in the opening, the cervical dilatation is 2 cm. or greater, depending on how wide the fingers can spread. As the cervix approaches full dilatation, an ever-smaller rim of the cervix can be felt at the outer edge of the fetal head. At 10 cm., no cervix can be felt at all.

As the cervix dilates, it is not only opening wider; it is also thinning out, or effacing. Before labor begins, the cervix is 2 to 3 cm. long. As labor progresses, it becomes shorter. This effacement is described in relation to the original length of the cervix. When it is half as long as the original measurement, the cervix is 50 percent effaced. When it is paper thin, it is 100 percent effaced.

Fetal station is measured by determining the location of the largest part of the fetal head in relation to the midpoint of the mother's pelvis. If the largest part is at the midpoint of the maternal pelvis, the station is 0. If the biparietal diameter of the fetal head is 1 cm. above the midpoint, the station is –1. As labor progresses, the fetal head descends into the pelvis, ultimately culminating at +5; at that point, the fetal head is at the vaginal opening. When your practitioner explains your progress, he or she will refer to both these numbers. For example, if you are examined after several hours of latent phase labor, your exam may show 4 cm., 0 station. Several hours later you may have progressed to 7 cm., +1 station. This means that in the intervening time, the cervix has dilated an additional 3 cm. and the fetal head has descended 1 cm.

If the cervix is sufficiently dilated, your practitioner may be able to determine the position of the fetal head. This is done by feeling for landmarks on the head. The bones that make up the fetal skull are separate and not fused together, as they are in the adult skull. The space between each bone is called a *suture*, which can be clearly felt between the bones. At the places where several bones adjoin, there are even larger spaces called *fontanelles*. The fetal head has two fontanelles, anterior and posterior, commonly referred to as "soft spots." By feeling the location of the fontanelles and the sutures, your practitioner may be able to determine which direction your baby is facing (occiput anterior or posterior, for example) and whether its chin is tucked on its chest.

In most cases, it is not possible to feel the landmarks on the fetal head clearly and accurately until the membranes of the amniotic sac rupture. When the sac is intact, the membranes overlaying the fetal head feel like a balloon, and the details of the fetal head cannot be discerned.

In early labor, especially if the fetal head is high, the cervical exam may be a bit uncomfortable. As labor progresses, the cervix dilates more and the head descends closer to the vagina. Consequently, each additional exam is usually easier for the mother than the last.

The Cervical Exam

The obstetrician or midwife determines three different things during a cervical exam: the amount of dilatation, the station of the baby's head, and (if there is sufficient dilation) the head's position.

After six hours of labor, this woman is anxious to hear about her progress. She is in the best position for a cervical exam, lying on her back, with her heels together and knees apart. She is somewhat surprised that this exam seems much more comfortable then the exam that she had on first arriving at the hospital. That's because of her labor's progress. Her cervix is now dilated further and the fetal head is lower, making it much easier for her practitioner to feel the head. In addition, many women start labor with the cervix tilted toward their back. As labor progress and the cervix dilates, it slips forward, making it easier to reach.

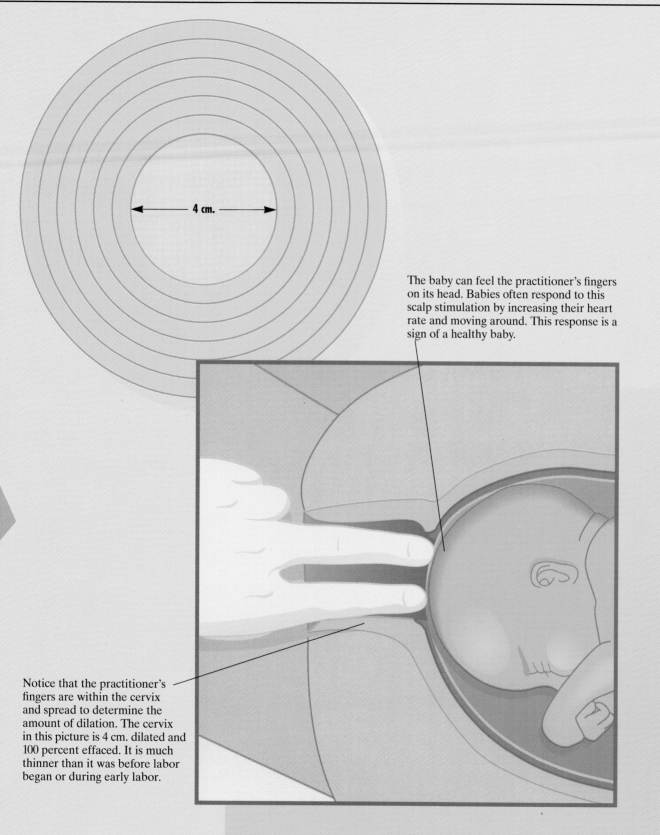

4 cm.

The baby can feel the practitioner's fingers on its head. Babies often respond to this scalp stimulation by increasing their heart rate and moving around. This response is a sign of a healthy baby.

Notice that the practitioner's fingers are within the cervix and spread to determine the amount of dilation. The cervix in this picture is 4 cm. dilated and 100 percent effaced. It is much thinner than it was before labor began or during early labor.

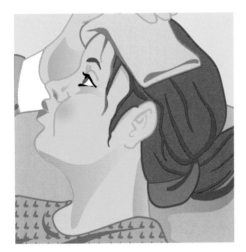

The Active Phase of Labor

YOUR PRACTITIONER HAS just rechecked your cervix. He or she tells you, "Seven centimeters dilated, and your baby's head is at +1 station. You're well into active phase labor." But you don't really need anyone to tell you that you're in the active phase, because you can sense the difference. The contractions are now longer, stronger, and closer together. When did that start? You can't remember exactly, but it must have been shortly after you noticed that your membranes had ruptured. So now, in addition to enduring the contractions, you feel fluid leaking a bit at a time. During the active phase, most women also experience uncontrollable shaking in addition to the pain. No one knows why this happens, although hormonal changes are undoubtedly involved. Amazingly, women who have *no* labor and undergo Caesarean section deliveries (perhaps because the baby was breech) also experience shaking when the baby is delivered. There is no way to stop the shaking; it's just a normal part of the active phase. Overall, things feel out of control, and you may be worrying. Is everything okay?

The *active phase* of labor is the second part of the first stage, during which the cervix dilates from 0 to 10 cm. As the name implies, this phase tends to be faster and more efficient than the latent phase. The contractions are longer, lasting from 60 to 90 seconds, and they are often more frequent, coming regularly every 2 minutes. Many women report that the contractions are stronger and felt more intensely as well.

In active labor, your body is working at maximum capacity, and it's easy to become overwhelmed by all the different things that are happening to you that are completely beyond your control. If you know what to expect, though, you need not worry that these very powerful sensations indicate something is wrong. Generally, they are a sign that everything is alright, that your body is performing this most miraculous of tasks with all the strength and ability that nature intended.

What might you feel? Well, first and foremost is the pain. There are a few lucky women who have painless labor, but the vast majority do not. Strong, painful contractions regularly occurring every 2 minutes and lasting 60 to 90 seconds characterize active labor. And they are enough to test anyone's endurance, especially if the active phase lasts several hours, which it usually does in first labors. During the active phase, many women rely most heavily on the breathing exercises that they learned in childbirth classes.

But some women find that the breathing exercises are not enough. This should not be surprising when you consider that breathing exercises do not relieve the pain, they just help you to cope with it. At this point, a lot of women opt for some form of pain relief, either a short-acting medication such as Nubain or Numorphan, which dulls the pain but wears off quickly, or epidural anesthesia, which stops the pain altogether by anesthetizing the lower spinal nerves. Both methods will be considered in detail in Chapter 24.

As the cervix dilates to 8–9 cm., the active phase becomes known as *transition*. This refers to the transition between the first stage, when the cervix dilates to 10 cm., and the second stage, when the baby is pushed out. Many women experience nausea and vomiting during transition, whether or not they have received anesthesia. No one understands why this happens, but it is a normal, if unpleasant, part of labor.

New sensations often develop during transition. As the fetal head descends, you may experience an almost uncontrollable urge to bear down or push. That sensation is going to be very important and helpful when it's actually time to push the baby out. Unfortunately, the sensation often begins before 10 cm. dilation is reached. Pushing before the cervix is fully dilated may cause the cervix to swell or to tear and bleed, so it's very important to avoid pushing until your practitioner tells you when you're ready.

The breathing exercises specifically designed for transition can be very helpful. You can't push when you are blowing! If you have opted for epidural anesthesia, you will not feel the urge to push. This can be a big advantage during transition, but it can also make pushing less effective in the second stage.

The active phase of labor is a very intense experience. As you feel engulfed and overwhelmed by many strong sensations, it helps to remember that these are the signs that your labor is progressing normally. Most importantly, they are bringing you ever closer to seeing your baby.

Active Labor

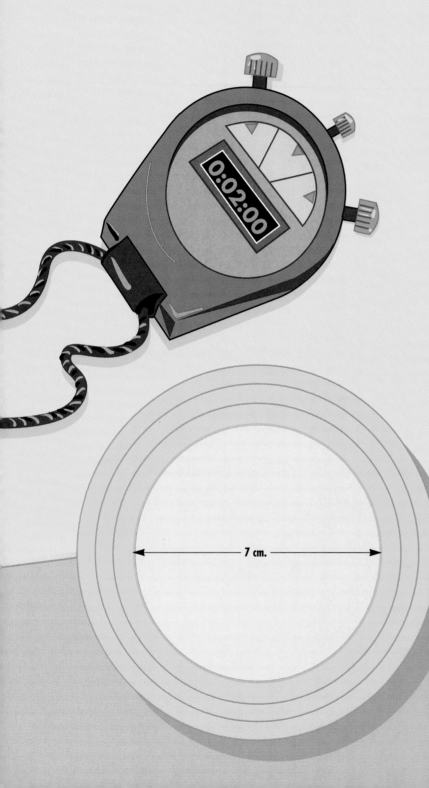

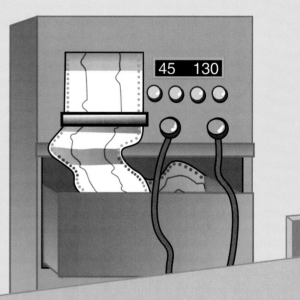

The active phase of labor is often more stressful for the baby as well. Even babies that are doing well should be monitored more often and more closely as labor progresses.

7 cm.

This woman's cervix has dilated to 7 cm. and she is in the active phase of labor. Active labor is a much more intense experience than the latent phase. Most women no longer feel like walking around and spend much of the time lying in bed or a sitting in a chair. Coping with the contractions takes concentration. The breathing exercises that you learn in childbirth classes can be very helpful.

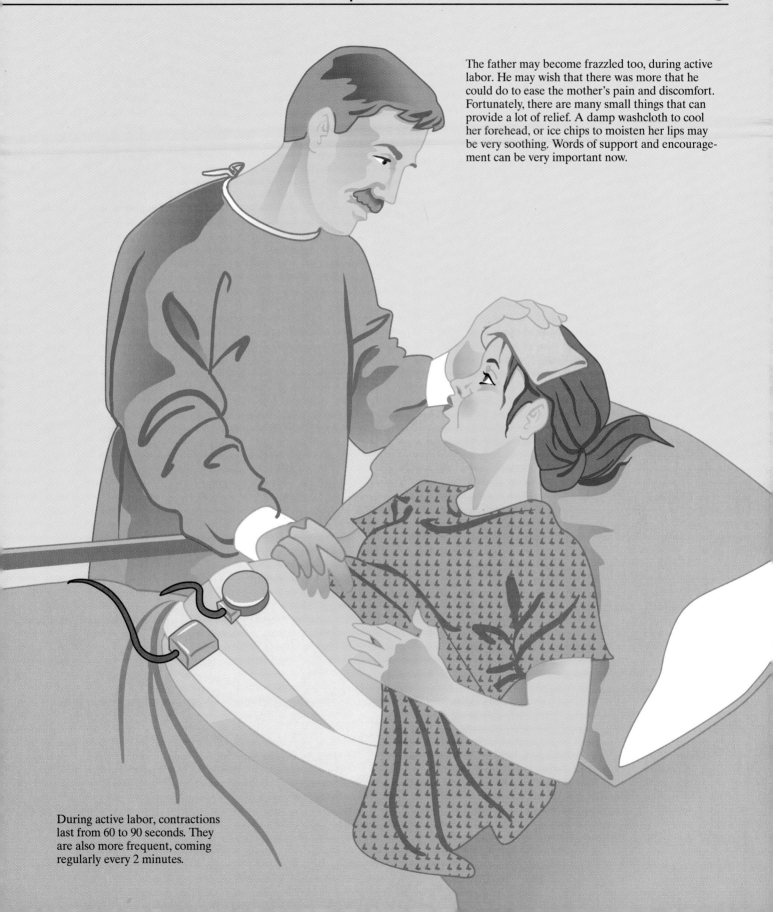

The father may become frazzled too, during active labor. He may wish that there was more that he could do to ease the mother's pain and discomfort. Fortunately, there are many small things that can provide a lot of relief. A damp washcloth to cool her forehead, or ice chips to moisten her lips may be very soothing. Words of support and encouragement can be very important now.

During active labor, contractions last from 60 to 90 seconds. They are also more frequent, coming regularly every 2 minutes.

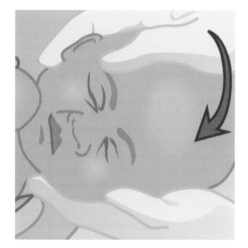

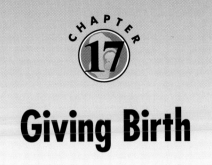

Giving Birth

Hooray! Your cervix has finally dilated to 10 cm. after 14 hours of labor. You may have thought that you were exhausted, but hearing this good news gives you a second wind. This is very important because the real work of labor is about to begin. It's time to push the baby out. Your practitioner may tell you that the baby's head is at +3 station. That means there are only 2 cm. between the baby and the outside world. *Station* refers to the actual location of the diameter of the baby's skull in relation to the midpoint of the mother's pelvis. The baby's head can be anywhere from –3 station to +5 station. The head achieves +5 station at delivery.

During the first stage of labor, as your cervix dilated from 0 to 10 cm., you were a spectator to the powerful forces that are unleashed in labor. The second stage of labor, in which the baby is pushed out depends on your pushing efforts. Although the uterus is still contracting approximately every 2 minutes, and pushing the baby further down, the most important force in the second stage is maternal pushing. This means that the harder you push during each contraction, the faster and more efficiently your baby will descend.

For some women, particularly those who have not had epidural anesthesia, pushing provides real relief. They may have struggled through transition against the almost unbearable urge to push. Now they do not have to resist the urge any longer and they can give in completely, following the natural cues of their bodies. However, other women do not find that pushing brings any relief. For them, the intense pressure caused by the baby's head as it descends just continues to increase the pain. Nevertheless, the thought that labor is almost over motivates them to push through the added pain and hastens the moment of their baby's birth.

A woman who has chosen epidural anesthesia does not feel these sensations. She may encounter a different problem, however. Because she does not feel the urge to push, she may not know *when* to push. She must rely on an assistant, such as the labor nurse or her coach, to let her know when each contraction starts, so she can coordinate her efforts. The assistant can tell when contractions are starting by feeling the mother's abdomen. In addition, some women experience a motor block as well as a sensory block when they receive epidural anesthesia. In other words, the epidural diminishes their muscle power even as it controls the sensation of pain. Although they may push with all their might, their pushing efforts are not nearly as strong as they might be without receiving an epidural. The fetal monitor can be especially helpful if you have an epidural, because you may not feel your contractions. Watching the monitor lets you know when they are starting, so you can coordinate your pushing efforts with the contractions. Pushing is effective only during the contractions.

This may pose a problem if there is a relatively tight fit between the fetal head and the mother's pelvis. The mother cannot push hard enough to push the baby out. That's why many practitioners recommend decreasing the amount of medication in the epidural, or even turning it off, in the second stage. Although there is increased pain along with the increased muscle power, it is often all that is needed to avoid a Caesarean section or a forceps delivery.

As the baby's head descends, the excitement in the room increases. This process usually takes from 1 to 2 hours in first-time labors, though it may be as brief as a few minutes if you have given birth before. Everyone can tell when the time for delivery draws near. First, the baby's head appears at the opening of the vagina during contractions. Then, as the head descends even lower, it remains visible even between contractions. You may experience intense sensations of burning and stretching as the baby's head fills the lower vagina. It's important to push past the pain. Sometimes it's hard to know exactly where to direct the pushing, and you can waste your efforts by pushing into your legs or against the bed. This position minimizes wasted effort. Also, opening your legs wide makes more room for the baby as its head descends.

In the second stage, the fetal monitor is used more frequently and for longer periods of time—sometimes continuously. That's because this stage is often the most stressful for the baby as well as the most demanding for the mother. Some babies may demonstrate signs of mild distress during pushing. Usually, supplemental oxygen given to the mother is enough to correct this problem.

There's no such thing as too much encouragement when you're pushing. It's hard work, and progress is often made slowly. Lots of love and support can make all the difference when your spirits are flagging.

When your baby is almost here, the practitioner will don gown and gloves in preparation for catching your new arrival. There's tremendous excitement in the room. Everyone shouts encouragement with each contraction. "Push, push, a little bit harder, a little harder!" Everyone is anticipating the birth, anxiously waiting. What exactly is the baby doing at this point?

The baby has just one more obstacle to negotiate. The top of his or her head must slip under your pubic bone before delivery can take place. With every push, the head comes down a little farther, but between contractions, it also seems to slide back a little each time. You feel the next contraction starting and summon all the strength that you have left. You push and push and push. There is a wild cheering. The baby's head has slipped past your pubic bone and is crowning!

Most practitioners do not decide whether an episiotomy is needed until this point. (See Chapter 21.) That's because it's difficult to anticipate how large the baby's head is and how much the mother's tissues can stretch. As the head is crowning, if the tissues of the vagina and perineum stretch to maximum capacity, and begin to tear and bleed, it may become clear that an episiotomy is warranted.

You feel tremendous pressure and burning, and the mixture of sensations is almost overwhelming. Your practitioner tells you, "With the next contraction, the baby's head will be born. As the head is being delivered, I'll ask you to stop pushing so the baby can have a gentle birth. Then I'll suction the nose and mouth so the baby's first breath will be easier." Once again you feel a contraction beginning and start to push. "Stop pushing," the practitioner calls. Your eyes are probably closed, but everyone present watches as the baby's head is born. The top of the head comes first, then the eyes, the nose and the mouth; finally the whole head is out.

The baby's mouth and nose are gently suctioned for mucus and amniotic fluid. The head, which has been facing the floor, naturally turns to one side. That's because the shoulders are entering the pelvis; they fit best if the baby is facing your side. Your practitioner then says, "With the next contraction, you'll push again for the baby's shoulders." Sure enough, the next contraction begins, as if on cue. The practitioner tilts the baby's head toward the floor and the top shoulder slips underneath the pubic bone. As the baby's head is tilted toward the ceiling, its bottom shoulder is born. "Open your eyes!" someone shouts. You look down in time to see the rest of the baby slip out.

Your practitioner either tells you, "It's a boy!" or "It's a girl!" and then hands you the wet and wriggling baby. The umbilical cord is still pulsating. Your newborn draws his or her first breath and cries out. You're laughing and crying at the same time. Your baby is here!

After the birth of the baby, the delivery of the placenta, also known as the after-birth, may seem anticlimactic. This remarkable organ, which has allowed you to nour-ish and support your baby for your entire pregnancy, has done its job, and must be discarded now.

The placenta is shaped like a pancake and is about 10 inches in diameter. From the earliest days of the pregnancy, it has been closely attached to the uterine wall. Once the baby is born, the uterus begins to contract around the empty cavity and, although the uterine walls are made of involuntary muscle and can easily become shorter and thicker, the placenta is incapable of changing its shape. As the surface of the uterine wall shrinks and becomes smaller behind it, the placenta begins to separate from the wall.

Blood vessels in the uterine wall that just moments ago carried blood to the placenta, begin to bleed into the space behind it. As blood fills the space, the pressure builds and more of the placenta comes away and separates from the uterine wall. This entire process can take anywhere from 10 to 30 minutes, on average.

When the placenta has completely separated, your practitioner will pull gently on the umbilical cord and the placenta will slip out. Although delivery of the placenta may be slightly uncomfortable, it is nothing at all like the delivery of the baby.

After the placenta has been delivered, your practitioner will examine it to make sure that it is all there. If you are interested, you can ask to see it, too. In most cases, the placenta almost always comes out in one piece. Nevertheless, it is very important to ensure that *all* of the placenta has been removed, because if it isn't, the normal uterine bleeding that occurs after delivery may be much heavier.

Postpartum uterine bleeding does not stop by clotting as most other bleeding does; uterine bleeding stops because the muscle of the uterine wall contracts and closes off the blood vessels. If any of the placenta remains inside the uterus, the uterus cannot contract completely.

Even after the placenta has been delivered successfully, you will still bleed a lot in the first few days after delivery; the blood flow will be much heavier than in your heaviest period. This is very normal and will gradually decrease over several weeks. Some women also experience cramping, known as *after-pains.* For reasons that are not understood, after-pains are usually stronger after each successive delivery. Often, women who had no after-pains after giving birth to their first child will have them when their second child is born.

If you are nursing, you may notice that after-pains begin each time the baby starts to breast-feed. That's because the newborn's sucking stimulates release of the hormone oxytocin, which triggers "let down" of the breast milk. (See Chapter 30.) This is the same oxytocin that stimulates uterine contractions. Breast-feeding actually encourages small contractions that stimulate the uterus to return to its normal size. Fortunately, after-pains last only a few days, so don't worry that breast-feeding will always cause uterine cramping.

Crowning of the Head

Your baby's head is almost *crowning*, which means the head is completely visible between contractions, and the birth is only a few contractions away. It is useful for the nurse and father to help the mother hold her legs back and wide open. This is an excellent position for pushing, because all the mother's power is transmitted to the baby.

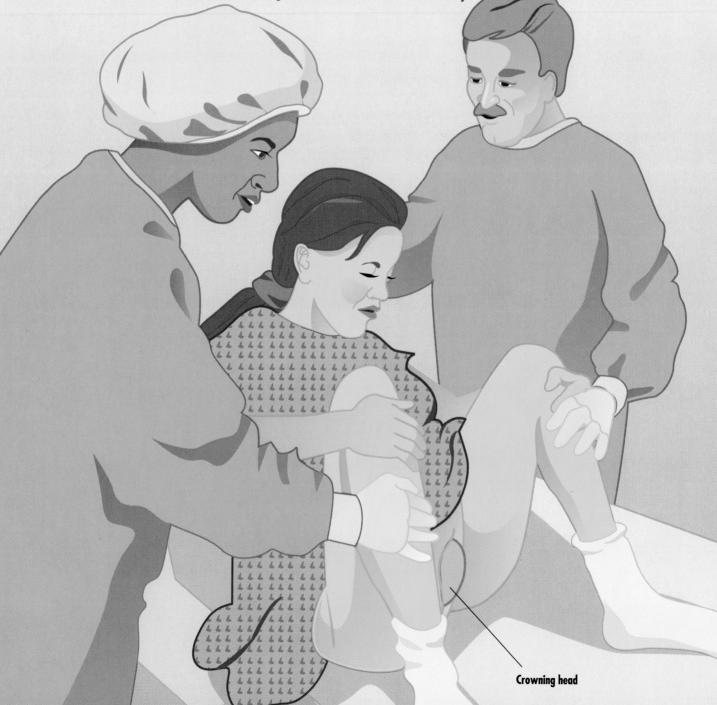

Crowning head

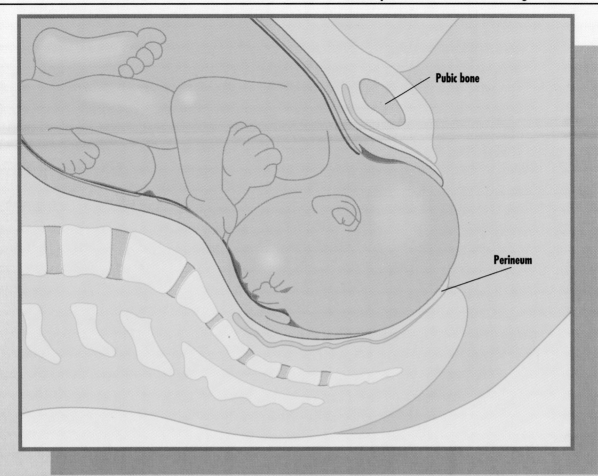

Pubic bone

Perineum

After almost two hours of pushing, the baby's head has descended to the vagina's opening. The last significant obstacle has just been negotiated; the top of the baby's head has slipped past the pubic bone, and now the head is crowning. It fills the entire lower vagina and stretches the tissues of the *perineum,* the space between the vagina and the rectum. This position is called crowning be-cause only the crown of the baby's head is visible.

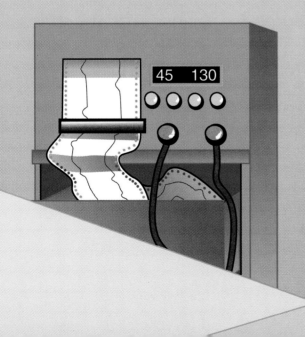

Delivery of the Head and Shoulders

1 At last, the baby is being born. This baby has descended in the occiput anterior position, which is by far the most common position. After the crown of the head has been delivered, the forehead is born, followed by the eyes, the nose, and the mouth.

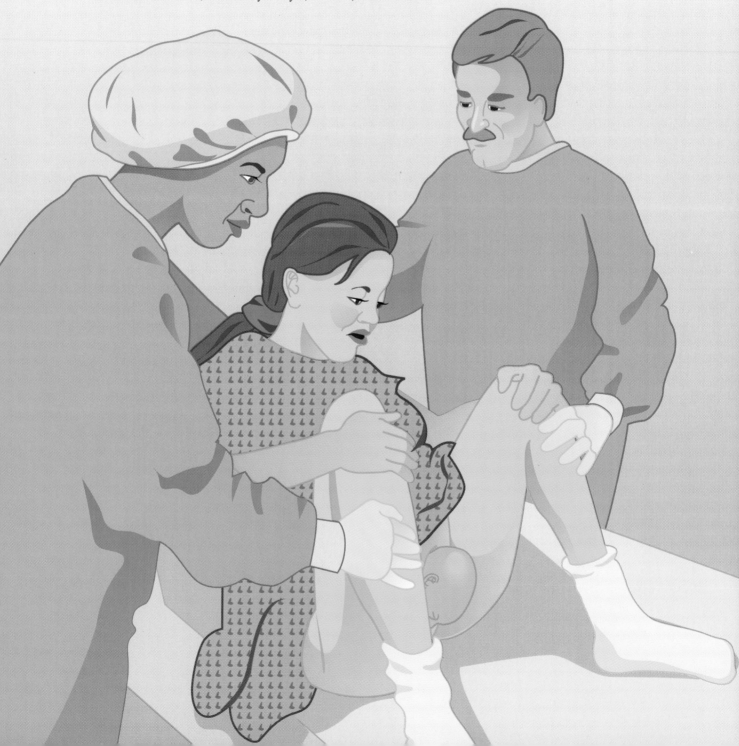

2 Finally, the entire head is out and the shoulders prepare to descend through the pelvis.

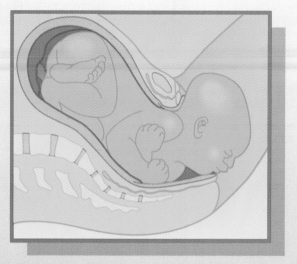

3 The practitioner gently suctions the baby's mouth and nose to remove excess mucus and amniotic fluid.

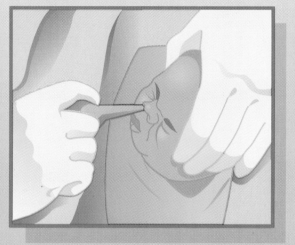

4 The best position for delivery is occiput anterior, with the head facing the floor. Because the shoulders are shaped so differently than the head, they must be delivered from a very different position. The widest part of the shoulders spans shoulder tip to shoulder tip. The longest dimension of the pelvis is usually front to back. Therefore, the baby's shoulders must enter the pelvis front to back. Now that the baby's head is out of the vagina, it is free to return to a neutral position, that is, with its head pointing straight ahead, relative to its shoulders. The shoulders must also negotiate the last hurdle of the mother's pubic bone. The practitioner can help by tilting the baby's head down, which encourages the front shoulder to slip under the pubic bone. After the front shoulder is out, the back shoulder slides out easily by tilting the baby's head back up.

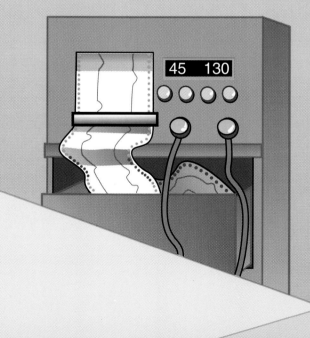

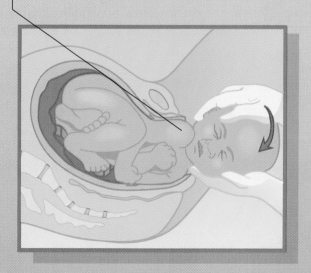

Delivery of the Body

1 With the delivery of the head and shoulders, the hard part is over. The rest of the baby slips out easily because it is usually much smaller than the head and shoulders. There are beneficial effects that result from the compression of the baby's chest and abdomen as it passes through the vagina. Amniotic fluid, normally present in the fetus's lungs and breathing passages, is partially squeezed out. Furthermore, the pressure on the chest may stimulate a breathing reflex, encouraging the newborn to take a first breath.

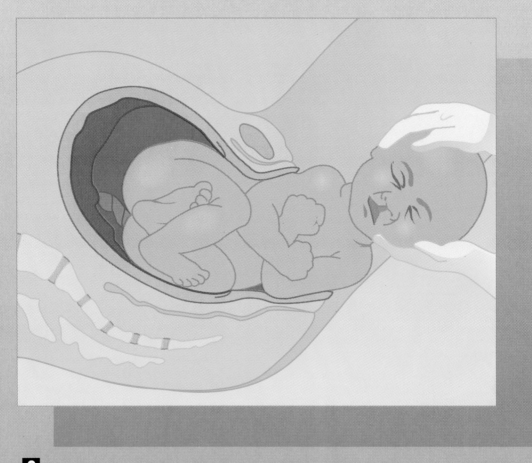

2 Your practitioner either exclaims, "It's a boy!" or "It's a girl!" and then places the wet and wriggling baby against your chest. The umbilical cord is still attached and still pulsating. Your newborn draws his or her first breath and gives a mighty wail. You're laughing and crying at the same time. Your baby is here!

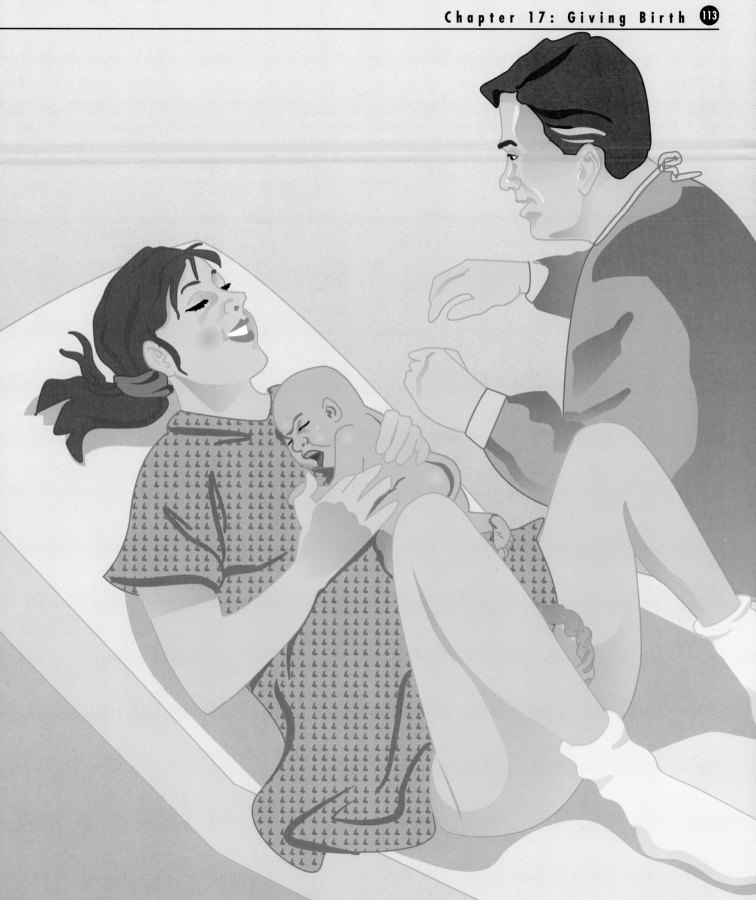

Detachment and Delivery of the Placenta

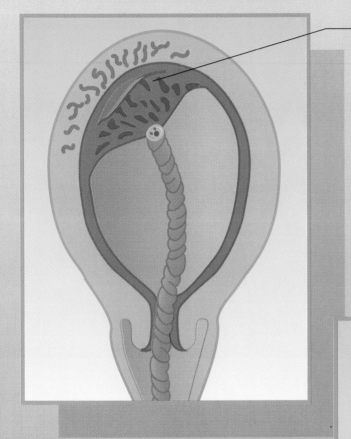

1 As soon as the baby is delivered, the uterine wall behind the placenta begins to contract. The surface area of the uterine wall decreases, but the placenta is not capable of contracting. Therefore, the placenta begins to pull away from the uterine wall.

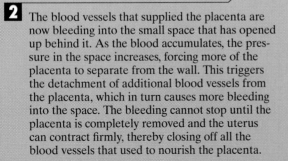

2 The blood vessels that supplied the placenta are now bleeding into the small space that has opened up behind it. As the blood accumulates, the pressure in the space increases, forcing more of the placenta to separate from the wall. This triggers the detachment of additional blood vessels from the placenta, which in turn causes more bleeding into the space. The bleeding cannot stop until the placenta is completely removed and the uterus can contract firmly, thereby closing off all the blood vessels that used to nourish the placenta.

3 With each minute that passes, more and more of the placenta detaches. Finally, the entire placenta falls away from the uterine wall. Gentle pulling on the umbilical cord allows the placenta to be delivered easily. Usually, the delivery of the placenta is preceded by a gush of blood, as the blood that has been pooling behind the placenta is released. Some women experience uterine cramping during and after delivery of the placenta, as the uterus contracts firmly to seal off the blood vessels that supplied the placenta. If the uterus does not contract firmly, and heavy vaginal bleeding persists, Pitocin may be given by injection or through an intravenous line to encourage the uterus to contract more efficiently and to stop bleeding.

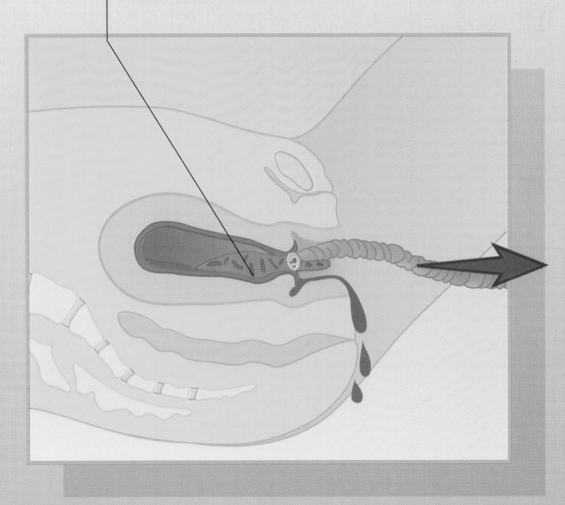

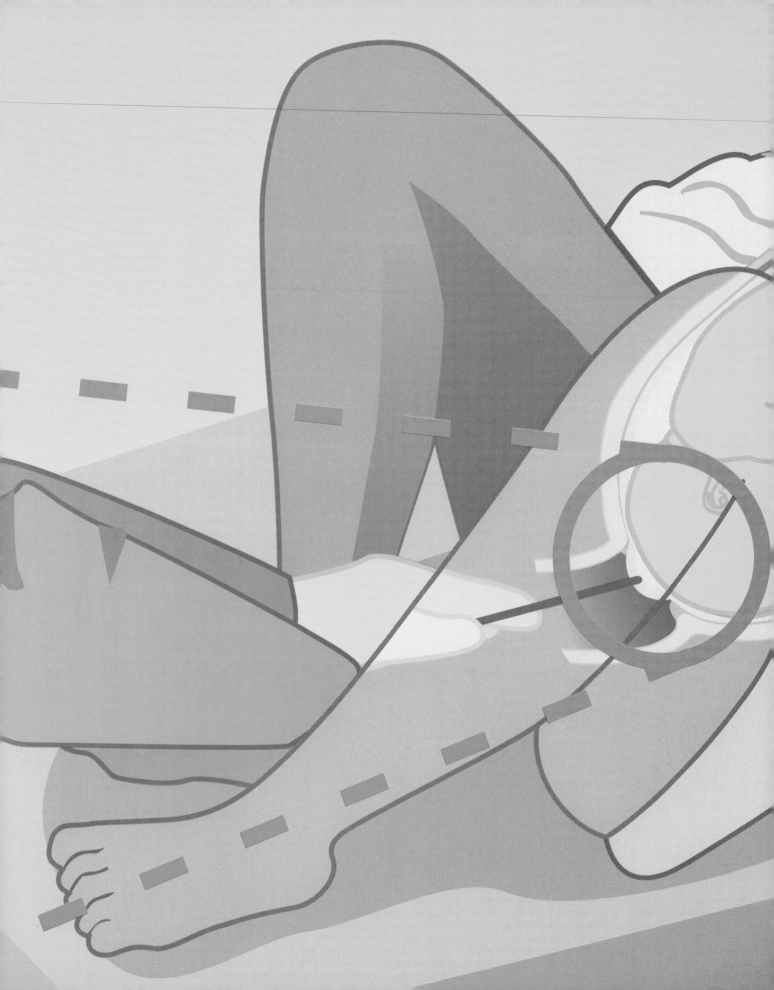

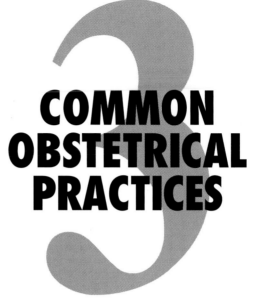

COMMON OBSTETRICAL PRACTICES

CONTENTS

OBSTETRICIANS AND MIDWIVES have become so successful at routinely delivering healthy babies to healthy mothers, that most people don't realize that this is a development of the twentieth century. In 1900, the death of women in childbirth was common, and virtually every woman expected to lose at least one child during labor and delivery. The practices and equipment of modern obstetrics have made all the difference in dramatically increasing the chances of a safe delivery.

There are proponents of natural childbirth without medical intervention of any sort. They contend that pregnancy and childbirth are and should be entirely natural processes. However, there is no reason to believe that just because something is a natural process, it is inherently safe. Think about it this way. While it is very likely that your baby will have a safe and healthy childhood, you are probably not planning to leave that to chance. You will take your baby to the pediatrician for routine checkups and immunize him or her to prevent dangerous childhood diseases. If your baby gets sick, you will not hesitate to use antibiotics, or whatever else is necessary to restore good health. The entire process of pregnancy through labor merits the same degree of close supervision and treatment, if it is indicated.

Modern obstetrics is based on the principle that most women will have uneventful labors and deliver healthy babies easily. Nonetheless, careful monitoring is done to detect those few babies that show subtle signs of difficulty and to treat them before a problem develops. Moreover, obstetricians are regularly called upon to rescue those babies that find it difficult or impossible to negotiate the birth canal.

Do obstetricians and midwives sometimes overtreat? Undoubtedly! That's because their standards are so high. To be sure that not even *one* baby will be harmed during delivery, it is almost impossible not to treat some babies that probably would withstand the stress of birth without help. To do otherwise is high stakes gambling. Most babies, even those showing signs of significant distress, would probably be okay without intervention. Some definitely will not. The average obstetrician or midwife is not a betting person; most won't take chances with your baby's health, even if the chances of a bad outcome are relatively small.

The chapters in this section are devoted to describing and explaining the most common practices and procedures of modern obstetrics. Each practice will be considered in detail, including possible reasons for its use, as well as how it works, and how it feels. Many of these procedures are optional in a lot of circumstances. That's why it's important to know as much as possible about them beforehand, because your practitioner will likely want to know your preferences.

In order to make a reasonable decision about what methods are best for you, it is important to be realistic about just how much pain is involved. The good news is that there are lots of options available for pain control—psychological options as well as medical ones.

Here, some particular comments are in order about childbirth and pain relief. Contractions are not called "labor pains" for nothing. They are not "sensations" and I've certainly never heard a patient characterize them as "orgasmic," though some books describe them as such. Although the pain of childbirth has been recognized in ancient writings dating back thousands of years, the following new myth about childbirth has become popular in recent years: Childbirth is not inherently painful, so "real women" don't need pain medication because they are actually "empowered" by experiencing the pain. But when you stop and think about it, this doesn't make much sense. A seven-pound baby is about to be pushed out of your body through a narrow (although elastic) tube. How could this be pain-free? There are a few lucky souls who may experience painless childbirth, but the vast majority of women describe it as the most physically painful experience of their lives. Whatever you do, do not plan too far ahead. You do not know how much pain you will have and you do not know how you will respond to it. Keep your options open.

In our relentlessly competitive society, it is often difficult not to set goals for ourselves, even in the most intimate of circumstances. It is important to remember that childbirth is not an athletic event. No team of judges will award the perfect score to the woman who refused an episiotomy, or deduct points from the woman who requested an epidural. Childbirth is a deeply personal experience. You should feel comfortable making the choices that are right for you; do not judge yourself by someone else's standards.

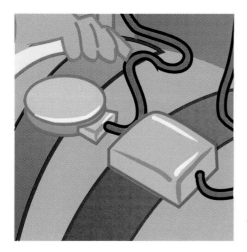

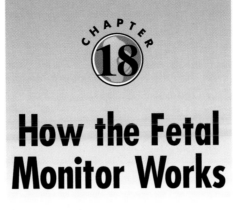

How the Fetal Monitor Works

USING AN ELECTRONIC fetal monitor is the best method of monitoring your baby during labor. It is the one piece of equipment that is routinely used in all labors, both normal and abnormal.

The fetal monitor looks quite impressive, but it's just a more sophisticated version of the monitor that your practitioner used to check the baby's heart rate at each prenatal visit. It operates on the same principle, using ultrasound waves to detect the movement of the fetal heart, and translating the changes in the waves to sound. In addition, the monitor can create a visual record of the heart rate because it contains a computer that instantaneously calculates the heart rate and displays the number. A pen continuously records the changing heart rate, producing a permanent graphic record. A second pen records the contraction pattern below the heart rate on the monitor paper. Monitoring contractions is very important because the heart rate pattern is almost impossible to interpret, unless you know when the contractions are occurring.

What do we learn from fetal monitoring? Monitoring the fetal heart rate can give valuable information about the baby's well-being, or health, in the last trimester of pregnancy. Also, fetal heart rate monitoring can be used to assess how well the fetus is tolerating the stresses of labor.

The *non-stress test* is an important method used to assess the condition of the fetus before labor begins. The name refers to the fact that when the test is administered, the fetus is not being subjected to the stress of contractions. A healthy baby, receiving an adequate supply of oxygen, will demonstrate a heart rate in the normal range (120–160 beats per minute). Also, a healthy baby is expected to move intermittently. This will be reflected by a rising heart rate that gradually returns to normal when the baby stops moving. Most babies who are receiving an adequate supply of oxygen will experience at least two *accelerations* (increases in heart rate) of at least 15 beats per minute above the baseline heart rate during a 20-minute period. These accelerations are usually associated with fetal movement. A healthy fetus who is receiving adequate oxygen will move frequently. An oxygen-deprived fetus will move sluggishly or not at all.

There should not be any *decelerations* (dips in the heart rate) on a normal non-stress test. A non-stress test is called *reactive* if the results are normal, an excellent prognostic sign. If the heart rate is not reactive, the fetus may be okay, but further testing is clearly indicated.

The process of monitoring the fetal heart rate in the presence of contractions is called a *contraction stress test,* although the test is done exactly the same way as the non-stress test. When interpreting a contraction stress test, two questions must be asked. Is the fetal heart rate reactive? And, how does the heart rate respond to the contractions? A fetus that was fine before labor started may have trouble once contractions begin to occur regularly.

The fetus who is receiving adequate oxygen across the placenta should not show any change in heart rate in response to the contractions. However, sometimes the fetal heart rate will decelerate. Not all decelerations are ominous. The significance of decelerations is determined by their relationship to the contractions—late decelerations cause the greatest concern. *Late decelerations* occur as each contraction is ending and persist after the contraction has stopped. Repetitive late decelerations are a sign of utero-placental insufficiency. This means the placenta is unable to supply enough oxygen between contractions to allow the fetus to "hold its breath" during contractions. Late decelerations warrant further testing if delivery is not imminent, and indicate a need for supplemental oxygen and other maneuvers that may increase the amount of oxygen available to the fetus. If late decelerations persist despite all efforts at treatment, emergency delivery may be needed.

Bradycardia, or slow heart rate, is another sign of significant fetal compromise. If the fetal heart rate drops below 100 for more than one minute, the dip is no longer called a deceleration; it has now become a bradycardia. A drop in heart rate lasting several minutes or more is, of course, cause for serious concern. If the usual treatment measures fail to correct the problem, emergency delivery is required. Sometimes a lack of oxygen causes bradycardia. Other less common causes of bradycardia include compression of the umbilical cord, or even a true knot in the cord.

Monitoring the Fetal Heart

Continuously monitoring the fetal heart rate externally is a painless and harmless process. Rather than having someone hold the ultrasound transducer in place over the baby (as shown in Chapter 4), the transducer is attached to a belt that is then fastened over the mother's abdomen. A pressure-sensitive gauge, attached to a second belt, is also placed over the uterus. The gauge detects the contractions and their relative strength and duration. Both belts are connected to the monitor's computer, which creates two visual displays: one for the heartbeat and one for the contractions. One pen records the changing heart rates, and a second pen records the pattern of the contractions on the monitor paper. It is very important to see both the patterns because the heart-rate pattern is almost impossible to interpret without information about the pattern of the contractions.

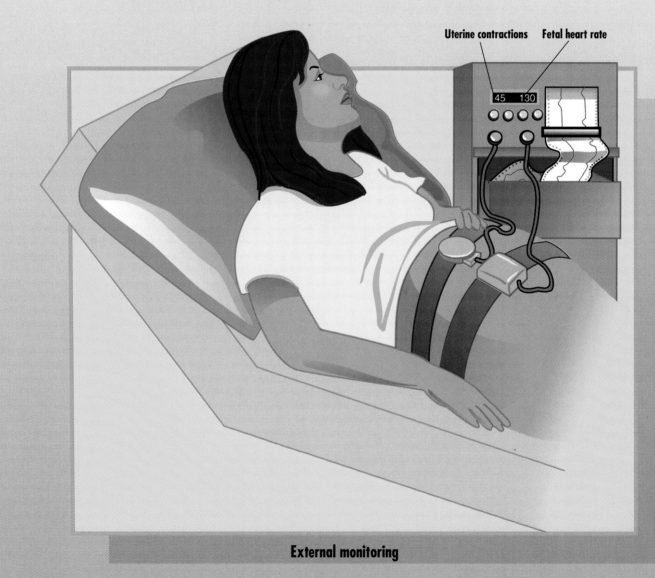

Uterine contractions   Fetal heart rate

45   130

External monitoring

The fetal heart rate can also be monitored directly, just as the adult heart rate is monitored during an electrocardiogram. Direct, or internal, monitoring may be necessary if there are signs of fetal distress, or if external monitoring does not pick up the baby's heart as accurately as it should. Internal monitoring is accomplished by applying a wire (the fetal scalp electrode) to the baby's head through the dilated cervix and attaching the wire to the monitor. The belt holding the transducer in place can then be removed. Once the fetal scalp electrode is applied, it must be left in place for the duration of labor. In contrast, the transducers and belts used in external monitoring can be taken on and off to monitor intermittently, as needed, during labor.

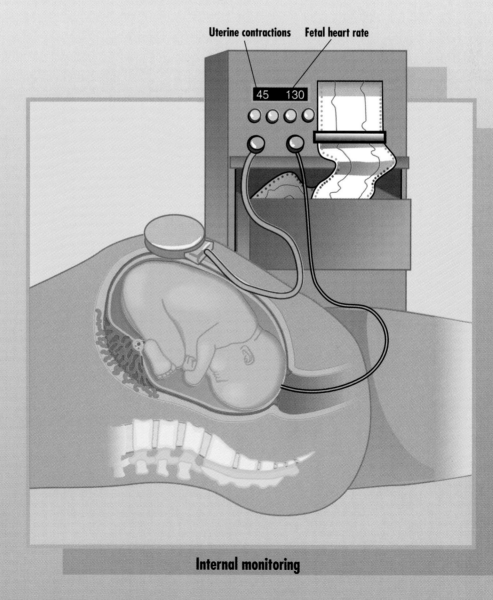

Internal monitoring

Analyzing the Results

The normal fetal heart rate is between 120 and 160 beats per minute. The heart rate of the fetus does not remain the same continuously; it changes in response to the level of fetal awareness, movement, and well-being, which is dependent on the oxygen level. These normal fluctuations are also characteristic of the heart rates of children and adults, whose heart rates may be slower and steadier when they are sleeping. Similarly, the fetal heart rate may be slower and steadier when the fetus is in a "sleep cycle." These observations form the basis of the most widely used test of fetal heart rate, the non-stress test. During the non-stress test, the fetal heart rate is monitored in the absence of additional stresses (such as Pitocin-induced contractions).

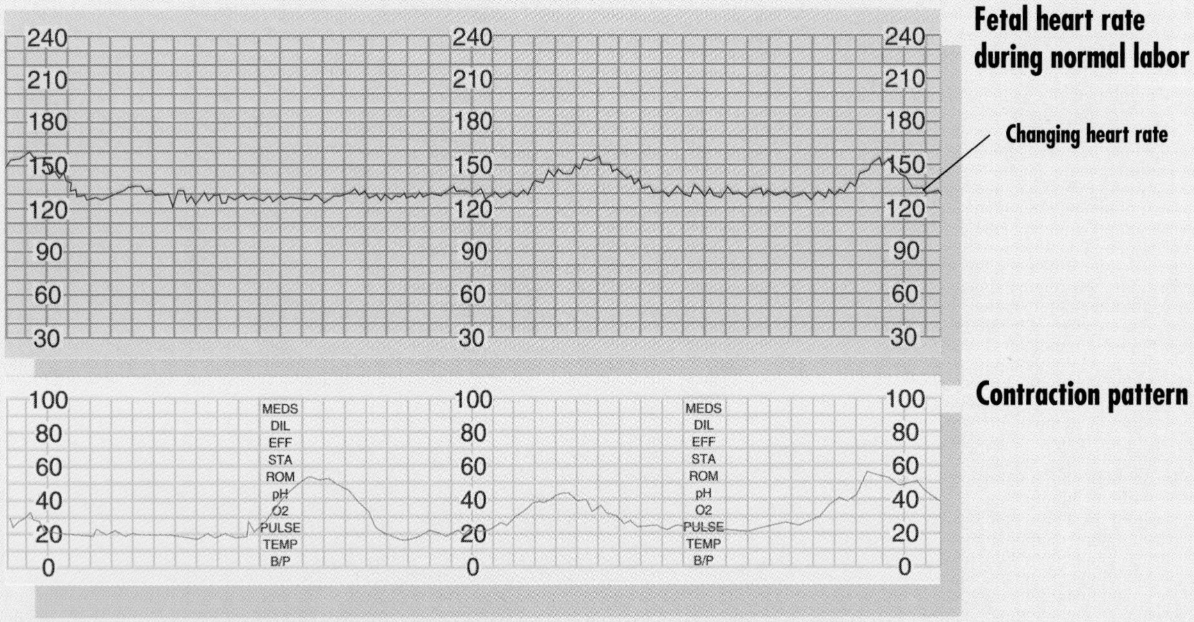

Fetal heart rate during normal labor

Changing heart rate

Contraction pattern

This sample monitor strip shows the tracing of the fetal heart rate pattern at the top and the contraction pattern at the bottom. The contractions are represented by the peaks in the lower pattern. This is a normal tracing, which reflects a reactive non-stress test. The heart rate is in the normal range and there are intermittent accelerations that occur when the baby moves. There are no decelerations in response to the contractions. This baby is tolerating labor without a problem.

Late decelerations

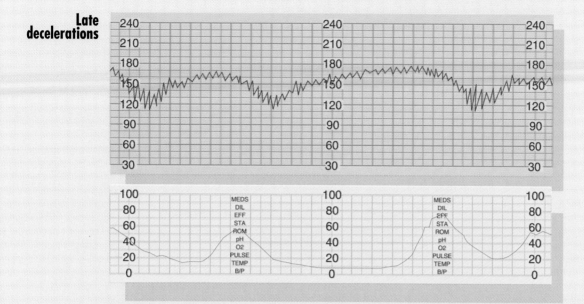

Compare this tracing with the one on the left. The most important difference is that here, each contraction is followed by a dip in the fetal heart rate. This suggests that the fetus is not receiving an adequate supply of oxygen. Although the heart rate is normal between contractions, the baby cannot "hold its breath" during the contractions. This is a sign of fetal distress. If this pattern persists, further investigation should follow to determine if the baby is capable of tolerating additional labor.

Bradycardia

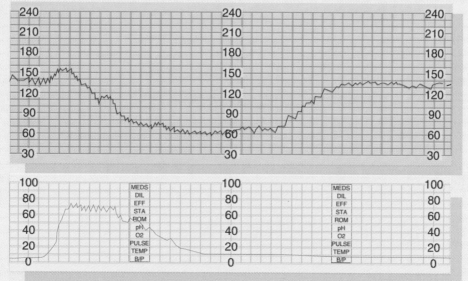

This is a very ominous sign. The fetus is so severely compromised by oxygen deprivation that it cannot sustain a normal heart rate. If the heart rate does not return to the normal range after the mother changes her position (perhaps the fetus is lying on its umbilical cord and interfering with the flow of blood) or after oxygen has been administered to the mother, prompt emergency delivery is required.

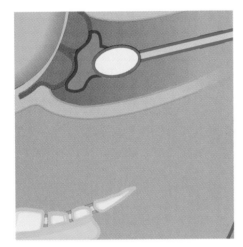

CHAPTER 19

How Labor Is Induced

YOUR DUE DATE came and went a week and a half ago. Your telephone rings constantly and every time you answer it, a friend or relative exclaims, "You're still home!" These last few days seem longer than the previous nine months. Your practitioner told you at this week's appointment that if you haven't gone into labor by next week, you will need to be admitted to the hospital so labor can be induced. Emotionally, you're relieved to have an end to the waiting in sight, but you wonder whether inducing labor is necessary and if it is safe.

Because no one really understands how normal labor starts, we are at a loss to explain why some labors don't start until weeks after the due date. This would not be of concern, except that after nine months of pregnancy have passed, the placenta often fails to keep up with the growing oxygen and nutritional needs of the overdue baby. In fact, the mortality rate of babies born after 43 weeks is double that of those born on time. After 44 weeks, the mortality rate is triple the normal rate. That is why most practitioners are extremely reluctant to allow pregnancies to continue much past 42 weeks.

Antepartum testing determines which babies are at highest risk for difficulties before and during labor. Most practitioners routinely recommend such testing after 41 weeks. It includes a non-stress test (see Chapter 18) and a biophysical profile (see Chapter 4) performed during an ultrasound exam. If this testing reveals abnormalities, induction of labor is recommended. Even if the test results are normal, induction is recommended at 42 weeks.

How is labor induced? There are a variety of methods, used alone or in combination, that can induce labor. If the cervix is more than slightly dilated, the simplest way is to rupture the membranes artificially (see Chapter 20). Most women will go into labor within 24 hours after the membranes rupture.

There are a number of disadvantages to using this method alone, however. First, not all women will go into labor. Second, as soon as the membranes are ruptured, the potential exists for *chorioamnionitis*, infection of the membranes and amniotic fluid. This type of infection affects the mother as well as the baby. The risk of infection increases over time. There is not much chance for infection to occur if the labor is well along and the delivery will happen within the next few hours.

However, if labor has not even started, the delivery may not take place for 24 hours or more, which significantly raises the possibility of infection. Chorioamnionitis can be treated with antibiotics, but it is far preferable to avoid infection all together, if possible.

The second method of inducing labor is the use of prostaglandin gel. This technique became available only a few years ago, but it has become popular very quickly. *Prostaglandin gel* contains one type of the hormone prostaglandin, which naturally causes the cervix to soften and thin out in preparation for labor. Prostaglandin gel may even stimulate mild contractions and, for some women, this is enough to start labor.

Prostaglandin gel is applied directly to the cervix during a cervical exam. Because of its potential to cause contractions, it is usually applied in the hospital setting and the baby is monitored for several hours thereafter. If no significant change occurs after four hours, a second dose of gel may be applied.

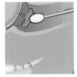

Prostaglandin gel may stimulate labor alone, but more commonly it is used in conjunction with Pitocin. Pitocin is the synthetic version of the naturally occurring hormone oxytocin, which causes uterine contractions. The advantage of giving prostaglandin gel first is that the cervix tends to become thinner and even slightly dilated after the gel is applied, making the Pitocin more likely to be effective at smaller doses. Pitocin is administered initially in minute quantities, and the amount is gradually increased over 20-minute intervals until contractions begin. The fetus is monitored during administration of Pitocin to make sure that the amount given does not cause the baby stress or contractions that are too frequent. If labor has not started within 12 to 24 hours after application of prostaglandin gel, the mother is readmitted to hospital to receive Pitocin through an intravenous line.

Are there disadvantages to Pitocin? Some practitioners believe that Pitocin causes stronger contractions than those that occur naturally. Most research suggests, however, that Pitocin-induced contractions are very similar to those of normal active labor. The potential does exist to cause contractions that are more frequent than naturally occurring contractions and, therefore, these contractions may be more stressful for the baby. That's why careful monitoring is essential during administration of Pitocin. It is easy to decrease the frequency of contractions just by lowering the dose of Pitocin if there is any indication that the contractions are occurring too close together.

The disadvantages must be weighed against the risks, of course. It would be inappropriate to induce labor just to have the delivery occur on a convenient date. The use of Pitocin for induction is justified only if the baby is at significant risk for serious problems, either because an abnormality has been found on antepartum testing, or because the baby is two weeks overdue or more.

There are other, less common reasons for inducing labor. These include pre-eclampsia, gestational diabetes (but not before 38 weeks), and intrauterine growth retardation (IUGR) if the fetus is in less than the 10th percentile for gestational age. In the case of pre-eclampsia, induction is performed to treat the mother. In the case of gestational diabetes or IUGR, the fetus is at risk.

Inducing Labor

2 A small amount of Pitocin is mixed in a large bag of IV fluid. The concentration of the Pitocin is known, and the quantity administered can be calculated from the number of drops flowing through the intravenous line per unit of time.

1 This woman is receiving Pitocin through her intravenous line to induce labor. Yesterday, she received two doses of prostaglandin gel. Her cervix, which was uneffaced and closed, is now dilated to 1 cm. and is 60 percent effaced. Although the prostaglandin gel did not start labor, the change in the cervix that it caused makes it much easier to stimulate labor with a smaller dose of Pitocin.

3 The intravenous line through which the Pitocin is running passes through this machine, which tightly regulates the amount of fluid that flows through it. In this way, very small quantities of Pitocin can be given, and the amount can be raised in very small increments.

4 Continuous fetal monitoring is important when Pitocin is being administered. The monitor creates a visual record of the contractions. In this way, the practitioner can be certain that the amount of Pitocin being given does not cause contractions that are too frequent. Also, the fetal heart rate can be assessed for any stress that could be caused by the Pitocin.

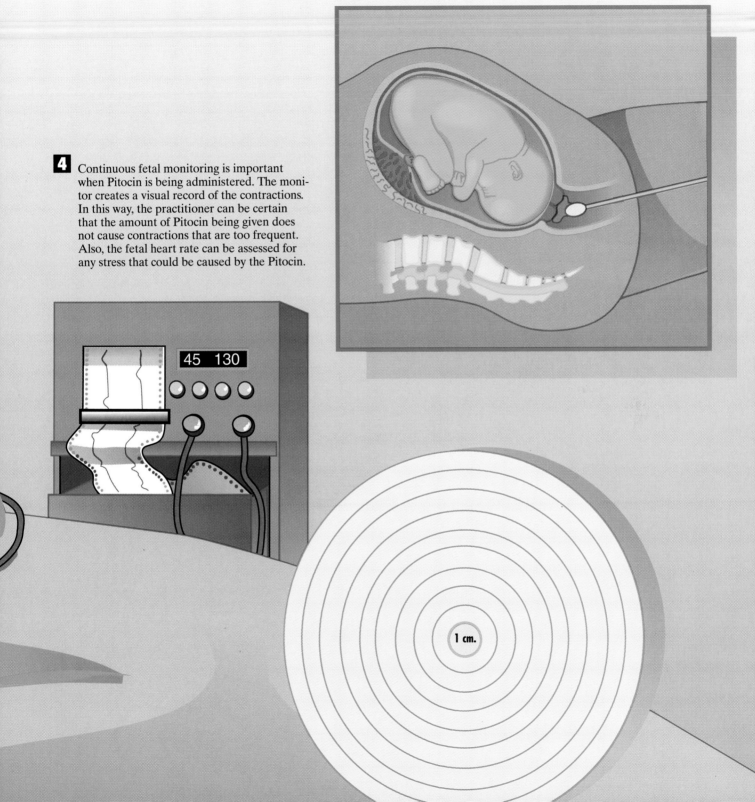

45 130

1 cm.

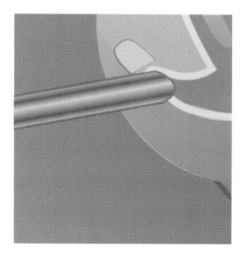

CHAPTER
20

How and Why the Fetal Membranes Are Ruptured Artifically

THE FETAL MEMBRANES protect the baby by forming a barrier to infection within the underwater world of the amniotic sac. The amniotic fluid cushions the baby from the bumps and bruises of the outside world. When the membranes rupture, announcing the imminent arrival of the baby, the delivery will take place within hours or days. Rupturing of the membranes is commonly called "breaking the water."

We do not have a very good understanding yet of exactly how or why the membranes rupture. Although natural rupture of the membranes is more likely as labor progresses and the cervix dilates, in some instances the membranes may rupture shortly before labor begins—even if the cervix has not dilated at all. In fact, in some women, the rupture of the membranes seems to trigger the onset of labor.

In almost every pregnancy, the membranes will rupture naturally at some point before the baby is born. In the rare cases that this does not happen, the membranes should be ruptured artificially. This will prevent the baby from being born *in caul*, which means the head would be covered by the membranes. If this were to happen, the baby would be unable to draw its first breath because it is still within the sac.

There are other, more common reasons why membranes may be ruptured artificially. The most common is to speed up labor. It is well-known that when the membranes rupture during the active phase of labor (either naturally or artificially induced), the contractions often become stronger and more frequent. Sometimes, this is all that is needed to speed up a labor that has been making minimal progress over many hours.

Another common reason to rupture the membranes artificially is if fetal distress is suspected. Rupturing the membranes serves two purposes: First, it allows the practitioner to place an internal electrode on the baby's head to record the fetal heart rate more accurately (see Chapter 18). It also allows the practitioner to determine whether there is any meconium in the amniotic fluid. Meconium is a sticky, green substance that is produced by the fetal intestine; it is the equivalent of a bowel movement. There will be meconium in a newborn's diapers for the first few days of his or her life.

The baby will pass meconium into the amniotic fluid in response to stress (such as oxygen deprivation). A small amount is not harmful, but a moderate to large amount is cause for concern. First, it suggests that the baby may be subject to stress by labor. Second, meconium can get into the baby's lungs, where it could cause breathing problems and even pneumonia after birth. If there is a significant amount of meconium in the amniotic fluid, a pediatrician or anesthesiologist may be asked to attend the birth and examine the newborn immediately, to suction out the meconium before it can be breathed farther into the baby's lungs.

Rupturing the membranes artificially is a very simple procedure. It is done during an ordinary vaginal exam; an *amnio-hook*, which looks like a large crochet hook, is used to scratch the surface of the membranes. It is painless for both mother and baby.

In many cases, your practitioner will offer you the option of artificial rupture of the membranes. In those instances, it is just a matter of personal preference as to whether you would like it done to speed up your labor. However, this procedure is advisable if the fetal heart rate tracing suggests the possibility of fetal distress. Rupturing the membranes artificially can provide valuable information for taking proper care of your baby.

Artificial Rupture of Membranes

The practitioner will usually offer the mother the option of rupturing the membranes when the cervix has dilated to between 4 and 5 cm. Notice that the mother is in the same position that is used for a routine cervical examination. The amnio-hook is scratched across the membranes, which can be seen bulging through the dilated cervix. It only takes a few seconds for the membranes to rupture. If the cervix is not dilated, it is not possible to rupture the membranes artificially. The rupture causes the baby no pain because the fetal membranes have no nerves. For the mother, there is no more than the mild discomfort associated with the cervical exam.

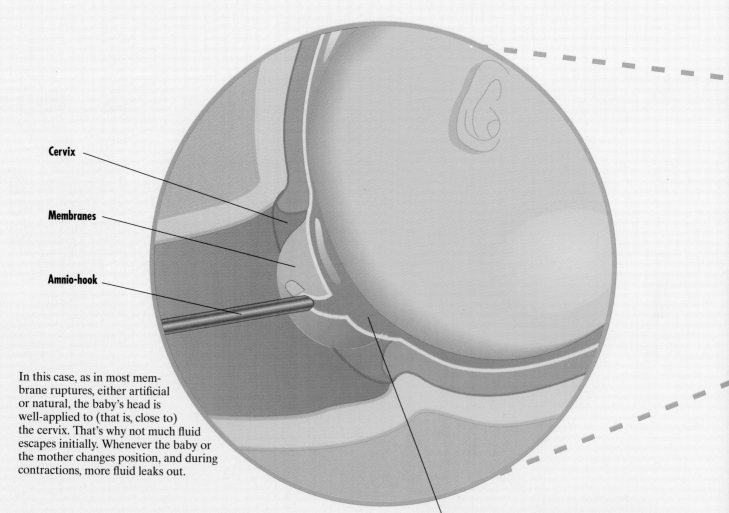

Cervix

Membranes

Amnio-hook

In this case, as in most membrane ruptures, either artificial or natural, the baby's head is well-applied to (that is, close to) the cervix. That's why not much fluid escapes initially. Whenever the baby or the mother changes position, and during contractions, more fluid leaks out.

Meconium Sometimes a green, sticky substance called meconium may be present in the amniotic fluid. It can be a sign of fetal distress. In this situation, the practitioner would evaluate the fetal heart rate tracing to determine the appropriate plan of action.

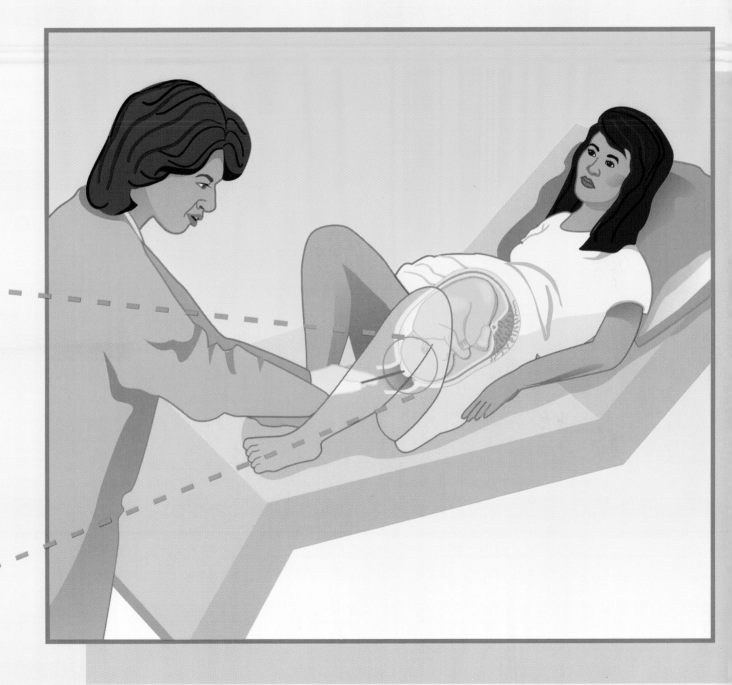

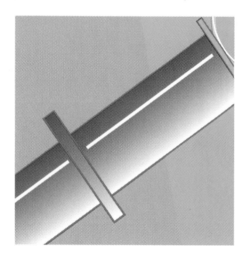

How and Why an Episiotomy is Performed

EPISIOTOMY IS ONE of the simplest and most common procedures performed in obstetrics today and, remarkably, one of the most controversial. It is difficult to understand why it is so controversial, when you consider how and why an episiotomy is done.

Episiotomy is designed to prevent uncontrolled, jagged tears during delivery by artificially enlarging the external vaginal opening. The area under the vaginal opening is anesthetized with a local anesthesia (unless the mother has already had an epidural), and a scissors is used to cut into the space. The cut can be either straight up and down (*median episiotomy*), or, if the baby is very large or the space very short, the cut is made off to one side (*mediolateral episiotomy*), to avoid damaging the *anal sphincter*, which is the muscle that controls bowel continence. After delivery, the episiotomy is closed in layers with absorbable sutures. There is no need to remove stitches later on because they dissolve and are absorbed.

Episiotomy represents the solution to an engineering problem: The baby's head is often too large to fit through the external opening of the vagina without causing significant tearing of the vagina and the surrounding tissues (these tissues are called the *perineum*). In some women, the external opening of the vagina will stretch to accommodate the baby's head. However, in most women having their first baby, it will not stretch enough to prevent tearing. Of course, tears can occur even if an episiotomy has been made, especially if the baby is very large. However, these tears tend to be extensions of the episiotomy itself, and are easier to repair than jagged, uncontrolled tears.

Whether tearing will occur if an episiotomy is not performed depends on many factors. Obviously, the most important factor is the size of the baby. A larger baby is much more likely to cause tearing than a smaller one. The speed with which the baby descends also plays a role in tearing. A baby that descends in minutes will not have time to slowly stretch the vaginal tissue, and tearing may result. Conversely, if you have pushed for many hours, the perineum may become swollen and incapable of stretching. This may also cause tearing.

These circumstances do not pose a problem for the baby or the practitioner; the baby will always come out. Midwives are capable of repairing most tears, and obstetricians are trained to repair *any* tears, no matter how extensive.

Vaginal and perineal tears have their biggest impact on the mother. Most tears occur downward, into the space between the vaginal opening and the rectum, and will stop short of the rectum. They are easy to repair. Such tears are similar to the opening created by an episiotomy. However, there is no guarantee that the tear will stop within the space. The tear may extend to the anal sphincter and this muscle may be completely ruptured by the tear. It is imperative that such tears be diagnosed and repaired on the spot, in order to prevent incontinence (loss of bowel control). The tear may actually extend right through to the tissue of the rectum itself. As you might imagine, such tears are much harder to repair, and the possibility of infection is higher. In addition, postpartum pain is also increased.

In some women, the tear or tears may extend upward, traveling near the urethra and possibly to the clitoris. These tears are not technically difficult to repair, but they may cause a tremendous amount of postpartum pain, especially after urination.

The decision to perform an episiotomy should not be made until the head is crowning. Only then can your practitioner determine if the vaginal opening is capable of stretching to accommodate the baby. A possible exception to this recommendation is if the baby is suspected to be very large.

Lately, it has become fashionable for women to refuse episiotomy. There may be no harm in refusing an episiotomy, but it's important to understand that the consequences may very well include even more stitches and more postpartum discomfort than an episiotomy may cause.

The Episiotomy Procedure

The crowning of the baby's head distends and stretches the tissues of the vaginal opening. It is at that this point that the decision about whether to perform an episiotomy should be made. Before crowning, it is impossible to tell if the tissue will stretch sufficiently or not. The decision should be based on direct inspection. If the tissue of the vaginal opening is beginning to tear and bleed, an episiotomy probably will be necessary to prevent more extensive tearing. Notice how close other important structures are to the vaginal opening. The rectum is only a short distance below and the urethra only a short distance above the vaginal opening. These structures could be damaged by uncontrolled tearing. Any tear can always be repaired, but it may cause a great deal of discomfort during the healing process.

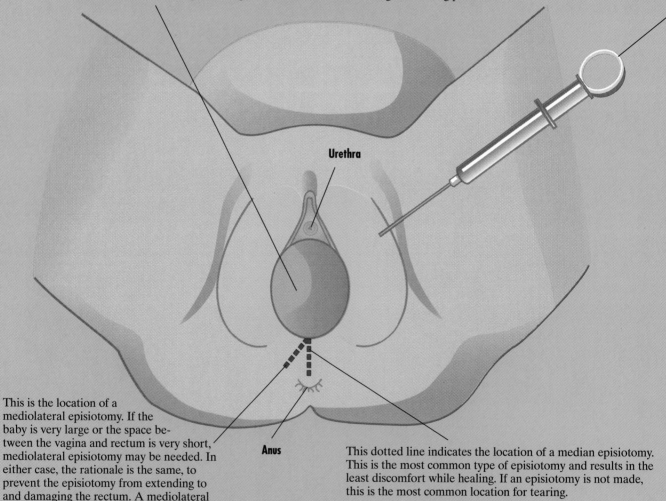

Urethra

Anus

This is the location of a mediolateral episiotomy. If the baby is very large or the space between the vagina and rectum is very short, mediolateral episiotomy may be needed. In either case, the rationale is the same, to prevent the episiotomy from extending to and damaging the rectum. A mediolateral episiotomy may cause more discomfort while healing than a median episiotomy.

This dotted line indicates the location of a median episiotomy. This is the most common type of episiotomy and results in the least discomfort while healing. If an episiotomy is not made, this is the most common location for tearing.

The practitioner may need to inject a local anesthetic to numb the tissue where the episiotomy will be made. If an epidural has been given, this anesthetic is not necessary. Injecting the local anesthesia may cause some burning or stinging, but this is usually lost in the pain of contractions and the strenuous effort of pushing; most women notice neither the injection of the anesthesia nor the cutting of the episiotomy.

The episiotomy is closed in layers using thin, absorbable sutures. The stitches actually dissolve while the healing is completed. Usually, there is not much discomfort associated with repairing the episiotomy. Additional local anesthesia can be injected if the original anesthesia wears off. After the anesthesia has worn off there will be some discomfort because of the stitches and the swelling. Ice packs do wonders to reduce the pain and swelling, and anesthetic creams also can be applied.

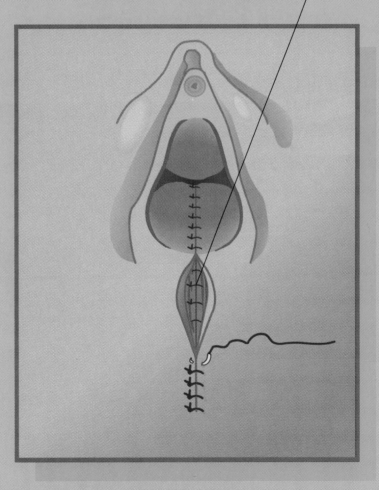

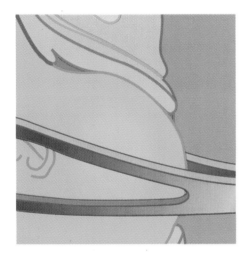

How a Baby Is Delivered by Forceps

I N THE MID-1500s William Chamberlen invented the obstetrics forceps, an instrument that changed the practice of obstetrics, or midwifery. Forceps were considered so amazing and so valuable that the Chamberlens guarded the design as a family secret for more than 100 years. During that time, the family became socially prominent and financially successful. In fact, when a descendent of the Chamberlen family was finally persuaded to sell the forceps for a tidy profit, he sold only half of the instrument, thus rendering it useless. Ultimately, however, the secret of the design was revealed and the lives of many women and babies were saved.

Obstetrical forceps were designed to solve the problem of the baby getting stuck in the birth canal, due to its size or position, during pushing. Using forceps enables the physician to pull the baby out. Until this century, when Caesarean sections, or C-sections, became possible, the use of forceps was the only technique available for treating this condition.

Forceps can be used only after the cervix is fully dilated and the head has begun to descend through the pelvis. If the fetal head stops descending despite good maternal pushing efforts, the use of forceps may be indicated. They are also helpful in situations in which the head has been descending slowly, but an immediate delivery is indicated because of fetal distress, or when the mother has become too exhausted to push anymore.

Modern forceps come in many types and are used in several circumstances. They look like large tongs. The two individual pieces (known as blades) are inserted separately into the vagina and guided into the appropriate position around the baby's head. Then the handles are locked together. When the next contraction comes, the obstetrician pulls on the forceps. These pulling forces, added to the pushing forces of the uterus, will cause the head to descend further. Often, several contractions are required before the head begins to crown. A generous episiotomy must be made to accommodate the baby's head with the forceps around it. The rest of the delivery is accomplished in the usual way.

The use of forceps is not without risk. Forceps can cause temporary or permanent injury to the baby or the mother, especially if they are used to turn the baby from an unfavorable position to a favorable one. As Caesarean sections have become safer, they are often recommended instead of forceps delivery because the risk of injuring the baby during a C-section is very small. This is one reason the rate of Caesarean deliveries has risen over the last few decades.

How would you know if a forceps delivery would be right for you? As stated above, forceps can be used only when the cervix is fully dilated and the baby's head has begun to descend through the pelvis. Perhaps you have been pushing well, but delivery is still an hour off and the fetal monitor shows signs of fetal distress. Perhaps you have pushed the baby's head down to +3 station, but it will go no further despite additional pushing. These are typical situations in which forceps may be recommended.

Unless the baby's head is very low (+4), there may be some discussion of a C-section versus a forceps delivery. That's because forceps cannot deliver a baby that is too big to fit. This is a common reason for the head to stop descending despite the fact that you may be doing a good job of pushing. If the baby is too big to fit, attempts to pull it through can cause serious injury. That's why the decision whether to use forceps must be made only by an obstetrician highly trained in their use.

If, after discussion, forceps seem to be your best choice, you will be given a spinal or an epidural anesthetic, if you have not already received one. (Forceps are large metal instruments, and placing them in the vagina would cause too much pain if anesthesia were not used.) Then, your bladder will be emptied with a catheter, both to provide additional room and to avoid injury to the bladder. If your bladder is full, it may be injured by pressure from the forceps.

It is possible that the delivery may not be accomplished even with the use of the forceps. If the baby is too large, or the position too unfavorable, the head might not descend even after forceps are applied. In that case, Caesarean section is the treatment of choice.

Babies born by forceps delivery often have temporary marks on their faces and heads from the instrument. These marks heal quickly and are no cause for concern.

It is important to remember that a forceps delivery is a medical procedure, with the possible risks that that implies. Forceps should be used only for a medical reason and not because you don't want to push. It is far better to push the baby out on your own than to have it pulled out.

Forceps Delivery

1 The mother is lying on her back with her legs in stirrups. Stirrups are not routinely used for vaginal births, except in the case of forceps delivery. Stirrups are helpful for two reasons. First, they ensure the proper positioning of the mother's legs to provide the maximum amount of room for the baby's head. Second, the anesthesia used in forceps deliveries makes it very difficult, if not impossible, for the mother to control the positioning of her legs.

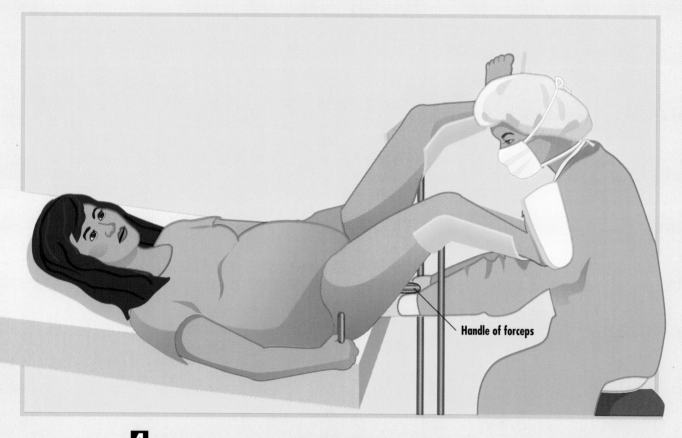

Handle of forceps

4 Depending on the station of the fetal head, the obstetrician often sits while using the forceps to ensure pulling in the appropriate direction. As the head descends under the pubic bone, the obstetrician may stand, because the pulling forces should be directed upward from that point on.

2 The forceps have been carefully applied around the baby's head with special attention given to the location of the forceps relative to the landmarks on the head, in order to avoid injury. The blades have been inserted separately. When the obstetrician is sure that they are properly positioned, the handles are locked together and the forceps are ready for use.

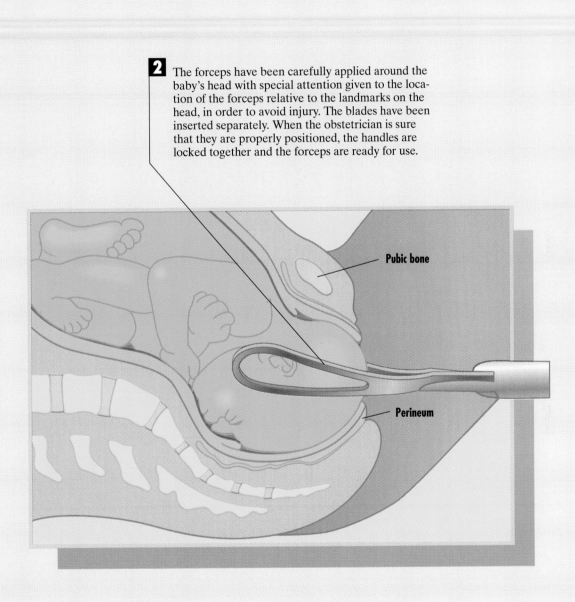

Pubic bone

Perineum

3 An episiotomy is not required to insert the forceps, but when the head descends to the level of the perineum, the combined width of the head and the forceps makes an episiotomy mandatory.

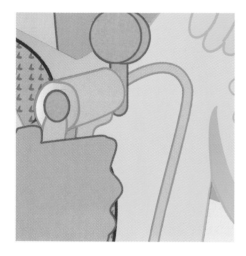

How a Baby Is Delivered by Vacuum Extraction

FORCEPS HAVE BEEN around for hundreds of years, and although they have saved the lives of thousands of babies and mothers, they also can cause injury. The obstetric vacuum was invented specifically to address this problem. It is an alternative to using forceps to pull the baby through the birth canal. However, unlike forceps, the obstetric vacuum does not compress the fetal skull, and therefore reduces the possibility of injury.

Obstetricians and midwives often joke that it is a shame that babies do not have handles on their heads to allow them to be pulled out when they get stuck. The vacuum extractor, which has a handle attached to a plastic suction cup, comes close to fulfilling this wish. In a vacuum extraction delivery, as with forceps, the cervix must be fully dilated, and the fetal head must have begun its descent through the pelvis. In a vacuum extraction delivery, however, the mother must be able to participate actively. When the vacuum is turned on, the cup sticks to the top of the baby's head, so the obstetrician can pull on the handle during contractions, adding pulling force to the pushing forces of the uterus and the mother. Unlike using forceps, it is almost impossible to pull too hard; the suction cup will just pop off.

There are advantages and disadvantages to the vacuum extractor when it is compared to forceps. In difficult situations, such as a higher station or suboptimal position of the fetal head, the use of the vacuum extractor has a lower success rate as compared to forceps. However, the vacuum extractor requires less maternal anesthesia, makes the mother an active participant in the delivery process by enlisting her pushing efforts, and is less likely to cause injury to the mother or the baby. Although there are some situations in which one method is preferable to the other, for the most part, the decision should rest with the obstetrician. The best method is usually the one that he or she is best trained in and has the most experience with.

In which situations might vacuum-assisted delivery be offered to you? The situations are similar to those in which forceps might be recommended: a period of pushing with progress to a low station, such as +3, followed by minimal further progress; fetal distress during the second stage (pushing); or maternal exhaustion. The vacuum extractor cannot pull the baby out without the help of maternal pushing. The same important warning that applies to the use of forceps also applies to the use of the vacuum extractor: If there is evidence that the baby is too large to fit, a C-section is the appropriate treatment.

What procedures can you expect if a decision is made to use the vacuum extractor to assist the delivery of your baby? The obstetrician will attach the cup to the device that creates the suction (usually a hand pump) and test it against his or her hand. Then the obstetrician will apply the cup to the baby's head and examine it carefully to be sure that it is properly positioned. At the next contraction, the nurse will pump up the vacuum and the obstetrician will begin pulling while you are pushing. Between contractions, the vacuum is released. The process is repeated until the baby's head is delivered. When the vacuum extractor is used, an episiotomy is not always necessary, because the cup is small and flexible; it does not add to the diameter of the fetal head. You can see that there is much less preparation involved than for the use of forceps. There are no special anesthesia requirements, because the suction cup is soft and causes no additional discomfort. There is no need for bladder catheterization, either.

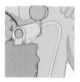

After your baby is delivered, you may be surprised and a little worried to find that the baby has a big bump on its head where the cup was attached. This bump (known as a *chignon*) is not harmful and will disappear in 24 to 48 hours.

Delivery by Vacuum Extraction

1 Vacuum extraction does not require the mother to have her legs in stirrups. The nurse can help her to position her legs properly. If the father or a friend is present, he or she can help with this, too. Often the mother has only minimal anesthesia because she must be able to push with as much power as possible.

2 The nurse is holding the hand-operated vacuum pump. At the beginning of each contraction, she pumps the device until the appropriate amount of suction is achieved. Between contractions, the suction is released, minimizing the risk of injury to the baby.

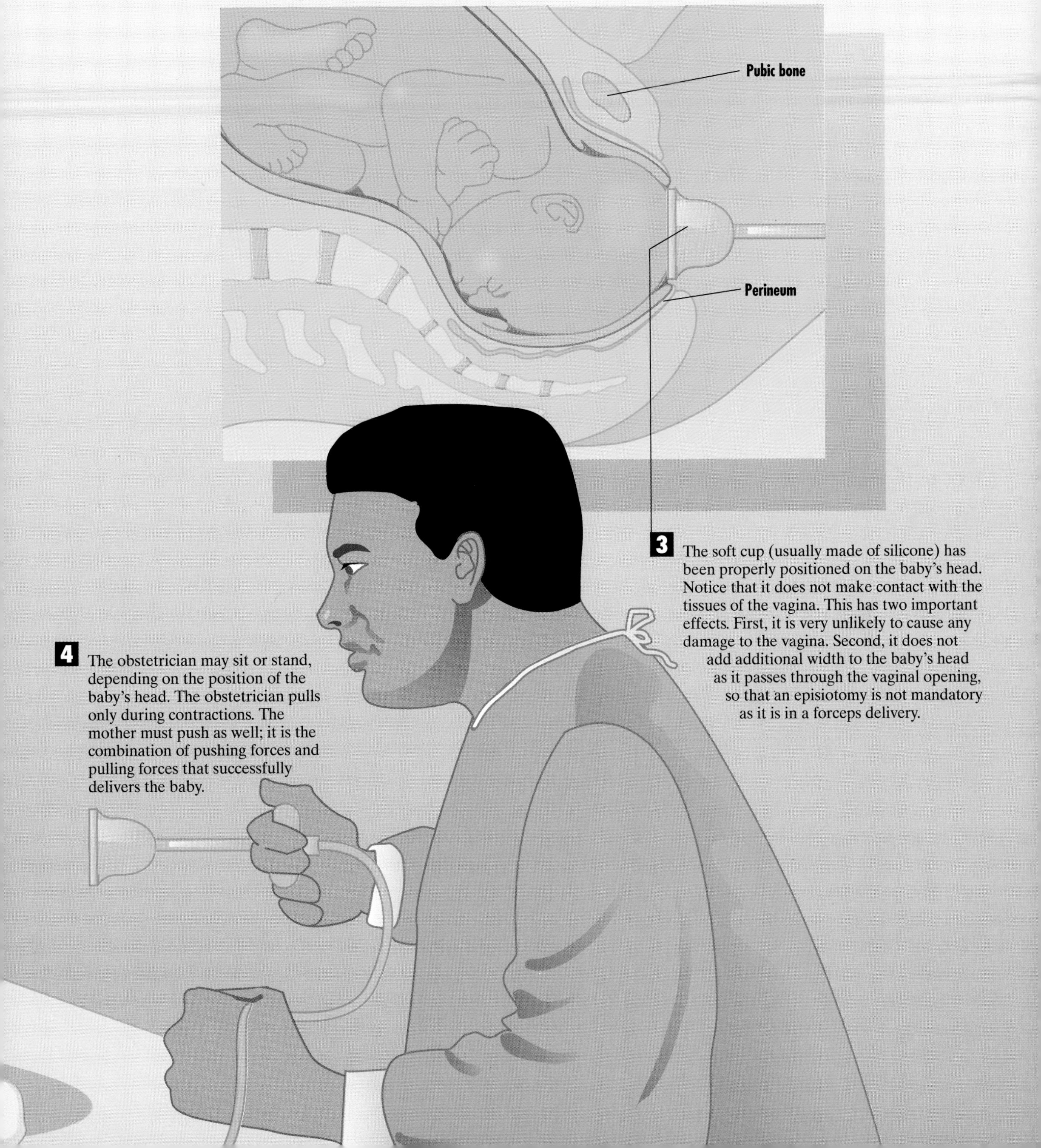

Pubic bone

Perineum

3 The soft cup (usually made of silicone) has been properly positioned on the baby's head. Notice that it does not make contact with the tissues of the vagina. This has two important effects. First, it is very unlikely to cause any damage to the vagina. Second, it does not add additional width to the baby's head as it passes through the vaginal opening, so that an episiotomy is not mandatory as it is in a forceps delivery.

4 The obstetrician may sit or stand, depending on the position of the baby's head. The obstetrician pulls only during contractions. The mother must push as well; it is the combination of pushing forces and pulling forces that successfully delivers the baby.

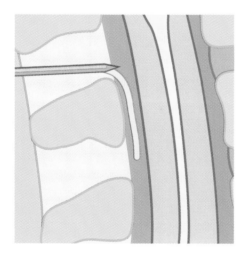

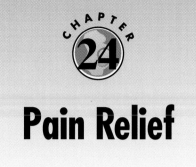

Pain Relief

THERE IS PROBABLY no area of obstetrics that generates more anxiety and more controversy than the subject of pain relief. That's not surprising when you consider the reputation childbirth has for being so painful. The truth of the matter is that the reputation is well-deserved. The good news is that there are many ways available to cope with or ease the pain. These methods can be divided into three basic types: psychological, narcotic, and conduction anesthesia (epidural and spinal anesthesia).

You should learn all you can about each of these types and determine your preferences. But do not make any firm decisions before labor begins. It is impossible to know beforehand what your labor will be like. Committing yourself to one particular type of pain relief, and no other, is a setup for disappointment. You may find that you need something quite different than your original preference, and you should never feel disappointed, or reproach yourself, if you change your mind in the face of actual experience.

Psychological methods of pain relief have come to be known as "natural childbirth." They were formulated in the 1950s as part of a larger effort to wrest control of childbirth from the medical establishment and give it back to women. Natural childbirth depends, in large part, on becoming knowledgeable about the entire process of giving birth. If you know what to expect, you are less likely to be frightened by this incredible process. Assuming that increased fear leads to increased pain, knowledge and preparation become your first line of defense.

Psychological methods of pain control involve focusing and relaxation exercises specifically tailored to each stage of labor. Most of these exercises involve specific types and patterns of breathing that are designed to focus your concentration on mastering the pain. Many women find that what they learn during natural childbirth preparation is all that they need to negotiate the long hours of labor. The advantages of natural childbirth include absence of side effects from pain-relieving medications and no slowing down of the labor process.

Unfortunately, to promote natural childbirth, some of its supporters have claimed that using the breathing techniques makes childbirth, at best, painless or, at worst, only slightly uncomfortable. Neither scenario is true. For the vast majority of women, childbirth is extremely painful.

Although the breathing exercises will help you to maintain control in the face of the pain, they will not relieve pain; after all, they are just prescribed breathing patterns.

Many women who are determined to use natural childbirth techniques often become frightened as labor progresses. The pain is so much greater than they have been led to expect and they fear that something is wrong, either with the labor or with themselves. Nothing could be further from the truth. Part of being knowledgeable about the process of childbirth is understanding how painful it is likely to be.

At a minimum, you should be sure to take a childbirth preparation course (offered by most hospitals and birthing centers) in order to prepare for labor and to familiarize yourself with the techniques of natural childbirth. However, if you decide that you need a bit more than natural childbirth breathing exercises to manage the pain, short-acting narcotics are often the first choice. These medications, such as Nubain and Numorphan, are related to stronger narcotics, such as morphine or codeine, that you might be given after surgery or a dental procedure. They differ in that they are much shorter-acting; they will be out of your bloodstream within an hour or two. That way, they are unlikely to be present in the baby's bloodstream at the time of birth.

Short-acting narcotics are given by injection, either into a muscle (like the buttock) or through an intravenous line. They do not take away the pain; they just "take the edge off." Some women find that this is the boost that they need to help them continue with the breathing exercises.

Because of some disadvantages that are associated with short-acting narcotics, it is preferable to avoid narcotics if the delivery is anticipated to occur within the next hour. Given too early in labor (that is, before 4 cm. dilation has been reached), they may slow down the progress of the labor. Narcotics cross the placenta and enter the baby's bloodstream, which has minimal effects before the baby is born. However, if the baby is born shortly after their administration, it could result is a sedated baby that is reluctant to breathe on its own. The effects of the short-acting narcotics on the baby can be reversed by administering an injection of naloxone.

For some women, neither natural childbirth breathing techniques nor short-acting narcotics provide enough relief. They prefer to feel no pain while remaining awake and aware. In the last 30 years, this preference became possible, with the advent of epidural anesthesia. *Epidural anesthesia* and its close relative *spinal anesthesia* are techniques in which the nerve roots of the spine are numbed with a local anesthetic. The effect is similar (and the drugs are similar) to numbing your mouth with novocaine in preparation for dental work. However, the numbing effect takes place over a much larger area, leaving you without sensation below the waist. Your labor continues, but you don't feel it.

Epidural anesthesia is administered through a tiny catheter (tube) placed in your back, overlying your spine. The catheter provides a continuous flow of anesthetic that bathes the nerve roots of your lower body as they leave the spinal cord. Usually, you receive continuous and complete pain relief. Sometimes, however, not every nerve root is reached by the catheter. In that case, you may have a "window," which is a small area that is not anesthetized. This can be very disconcerting, but it can usually be fixed by readjusting the catheter.

The advantages of an epidural are obvious: You can experience a pain-free labor while remaining awake and fully aware. There are disadvantages, though, and these are not trivial. Epidural anesthesia, if given too early in labor (before 4 cm. dilation) can slow the progress of labor significantly, often so much so that an intervention that will strengthen the contractions, such as Pitocin, is required. Epidural anesthesia can also anesthetize the nerves that control the diameter of blood vessels and thereby regulate blood pressure. After an epidural is administered, you may experience a temporary drop in blood pressure, which may decrease blood flow to the baby. This condition can be corrected with extra intravenous fluid or medication, if necessary.

Finally, an epidural can also anesthetize the nerves that control muscles, which may hamper your ability to push when the time comes. If the baby is small and your pelvis is large, this will be of no consequence; you will be able to push the baby out anyway. But if the fit is tight, this diminution of your strength may make it very difficult to push the baby out.

The rate of forceps and vacuum-assisted deliveries is much higher in women who have received epidural anesthesia, due to the temporary loss of muscular strength. Because the amount of anesthetic flowing through the catheter can be regulated, if the amount is lowered, you will regain some or all of your muscle strength. Of course, you will also regain some pain. The trade-off, then, is increased pain for increased muscle power. If you are anxious to avoid forceps or vacuum, this may be the right trade-off for you.

Spinal anesthesia operates on the same principle as epidural anesthesia and was often used in labor before epidurals became available. Because of its distinct characteristics, spinal anesthesia is now considered more appropriate for C-sections and forceps deliveries than for labor. Spinal anesthesia requires the injection of anesthetic directly into the space surrounding the spinal cord. It is administered in the same way as an epidural, but no catheter is left in place. Because only a one-time dose can be given, the amount of anesthetic injected in relatively large. This results in quick (5 minutes versus 15 for epidural) action and dense (strong) anesthesia. The anesthetic almost always affects motor nerves, and therefore muscle power, significantly. Most women lose control over their legs and cannot push effectively after a spinal anesthetic has been given.These qualities present severe disadvantages in labor, but make spinals especially useful during C-sections. They provide quick anesthesia, strong enough to allow major abdominal surgery with no pain at all. Best of all, the mother is awake and aware throughout the surgery.

Today, there are a wide variety of options available for pain relief in labor. Consider them all, and try to determine your preference, but wait until you actually experience labor before making the decision that is right for you. Above all, do not be frightened or disappointed if you find that labor is more painful than you anticipated, and that you need pain medication you thought you would avoid. Experience is still, after all, the best teacher.

Placement of an Epidural

1 The best position for administering an epidural requires the mother to lie on her side. The nurse is helping her to curl the rest of her body around the baby. This position pushes the mother's back toward the anesthesiologist who is sitting behind her.

3 The anesthesiologist has just passed the catheter into the epidural space and removed the needle. Notice that the mother's back has been draped as if for a surgical procedure. It is very important to maintain sterile conditions while the epidural catheter is being inserted. The anesthesiologist will then tape the catheter in place, so the mother can move without fear of dislodging it.

2 An epidural is most often administered by an anesthesiologist. The anesthesiologist begins by examining the mother's back to find the most favorable space between the vertebrae to insert the catheter. Once the best location has been identified, the anesthesiologist numbs the overlying skin with a small amount of local anesthetic. A needle is inserted and carefully advanced into the epidural space (the space outside the covering of the spinal cord). Then the catheter is passed through the needle into the epidural space and the needle is removed.

4 The anesthetic passes through this very thin catheter into the epidural space bathing all the nerve roots below the level of the catheter. Within 10–15 minutes after beginning the anesthetic infusion, the mother should feel relief from the pain.

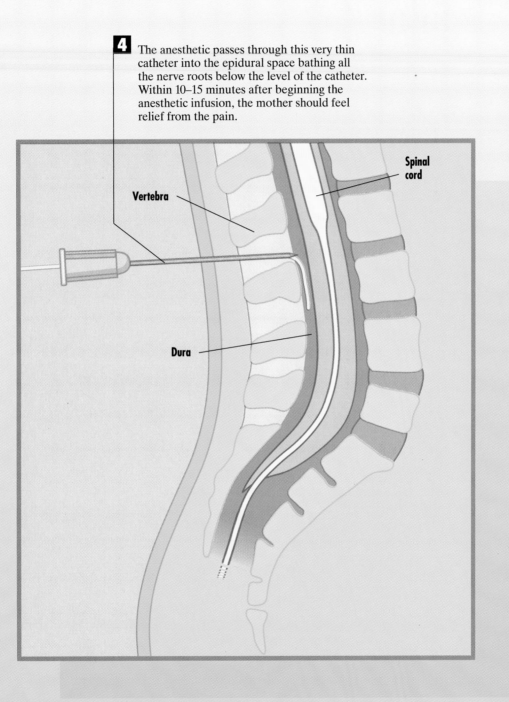

5 This drawing shows the layers between the skin of the back and the spinal cord. Notice that the epidural catheter is placed in the epidural space, and it remains outside of the covering of the spinal cord.

Placement of Spinal Anesthesia

1 Spinal anesthestics are usually administered by anesthesiologists, although in some parts of the country, obstetricians are also trained to administer them.

2 This woman is sitting while the spinal anesthetic is inserted. Spinal anesthetics can also be administered while the mother lies on her side. As with the epidural, the anesthesiologist chooses the position based on which position provides the best approach to the spot where the needle will be inserted. She is curling over the baby, and placing her chin on her chest in order to push her back out.

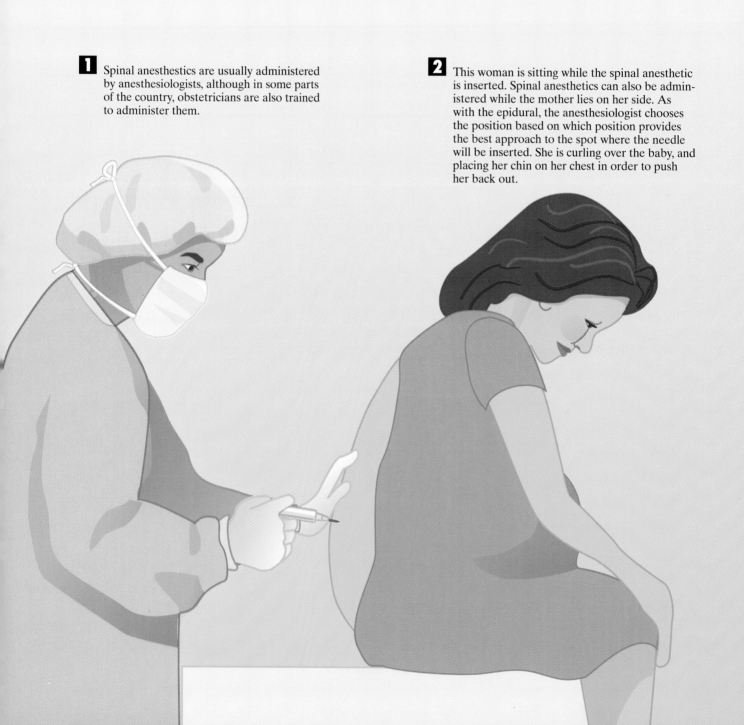

3 This procedure is also done under sterile conditions. As with an epidural, the overlying skin is first anesthetized with a small amount of local anesthetic. Then, a very thin needle is passed through the covering of the spinal cord (the *dura*) into the space around the cord itself. The anesthetic is injected directly through the needle and the needle is then removed. No catheter is left in place. A very thin needle is used to minimize the size of the hole left in the dura. A hole that is too large will not seal quickly, and some spinal fluid may escape. This can cause a "spinal headache" for hours after the delivery. Spinal headaches occur after less than 1 percent of all spinals. Usually, a spinal headache will resolve by itself. Only in rare instances is any further treatment required.

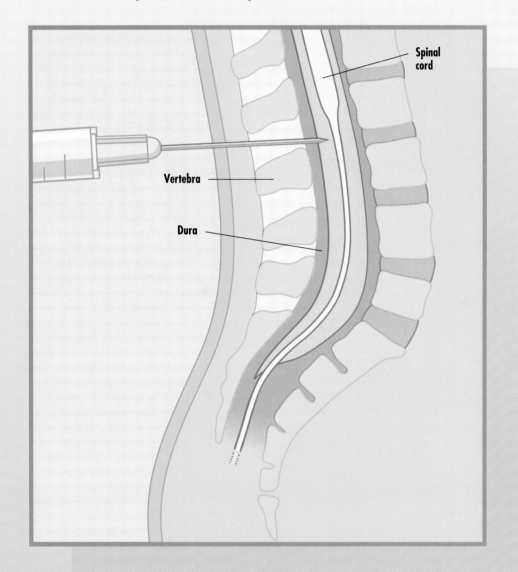

4 Compare this picture of the mother's back to the enlargment that accompanies the illustration for an epidural. Notice that the needle passes through the epidural space and through the dura covering the spinal cord. The anesthetic that is injected through the needle bathes the spinal cord itself.

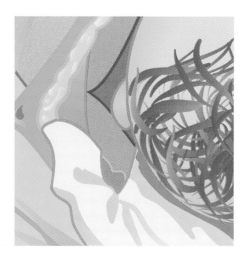

CHAPTER 25

How a Baby is Delivered by Caesarean Section

AMID ALL THE negative publicity about the rising rate of Caesarean sections, it is easy to lose sight of the fact that it is often a life-saving operation. Literally tens of thousands, and perhaps hundreds of thousands, of babies and mothers are saved each year. The Caesarean section is probably the single most important factor responsible for the dramatically lower rates of maternal and neonatal deaths since the beginning of this century (and medical advances have made it safer now than ever before).

Nonetheless, it is possible to have too much of a good thing. The odds are as high as 1 in 5 that Caesarean section will be recommended to you. How will you know if it is the right procedure for your situation? How can you avoid having an unnecessary Caesarean section? The first step toward answering both questions is to understand exactly what a Caesarean section is—and when it is recommended.

Caesarean section is the operation in which a baby is delivered through an incision in the abdomen, rather than through the vagina. It is named after Julius Caesar; as legend has it, he was born this way. It is often referred to as C-section.

The most common reason for a C-section is *cephalopelvic disproportion* (CPD), which is just a complicated way of saying that the baby's head does not fit through the mother's pelvis. This can happen for a variety of reasons, including an unusually large baby, an unusually small pelvis, or an unusual position of the baby, such as occiput posterior presentation. CPD is a diagnosis that can be made only during labor. If the labor fails to progress beyond a certain point, despite good contractions for a least two hours (often strengthened by Pitocin), it is unlikely that the baby is going to fit.

You might imagine that every labor would automatically progress to 10 cm. dilation and that the difficulty would arise during the attempt to push the baby out. However, in some way that we do not yet understand, the uterus senses that the baby cannot fit properly. Cervical dilation may stop several centimeters before full dilation, and no further progress will be made despite many additional hours of labor. Whether progress stops in the active phase or during pushing, it is a sign that C-section may be necessary. Without full dilation of the cervix, C-section is the only option; if progress stops during pushing, forceps or vacuum extraction may be considered if the baby's head is low enough.

There are undoubtedly some unnecessary C-sections that are done presumably because of CPD. It is important for the practitioner to wait until the active phase before making the decision that the baby cannot fit. In the latent, or first, phase of labor, progress may be extremely slow and may take many hours; this is a sign that labor hasn't really started efficiently, not a sign that the baby doesn't fit. As a general rule, the diagnosis of CPD should not be made before approximately 5 cm. dilation.

Another contributing factor to unnecessary C-sections for CPD is pain relief that is given too early. Short-acting narcotics and epidural anesthesia sometimes interfere with the progress of labor before the active phase begins. If you are anxious to avoid a C-section, it is best to wait until 4–5 cm. dilation before asking for pain relief.

Additionally, a large number of C-sections are done for breech presentation. As discussed in detail in Chapters 12, 26, and 27, vaginal delivery from the breech presentation involves much greater risk than vaginal delivery head first. If attempts to turn the baby have been unsuccessful, C-section is often recommended. In this situation, most women, wishing to minimize *any* risk to the baby, select C-section as the preferred delivery option. However, most C-sections done for breech presentation could be considered unnecessary in the sense that vaginal delivery of most breech babies turns out fine. Unfortunately, at present we have no way of determining with any certainty which breech babies will be permanently injured by vaginal delivery.

Another common reason for C-section deliveries, and probably the most controversial, is fetal distress. These C-sections are performed because the practitioner suspects that the baby is being deprived of oxygen. The diagnosis is usually made by analyzing the fetal heart rate tracing, although other factors such as moderate to thick meconium in the amniotic fluid can raise suspicions or lend support to the diagnosis. More sophisticated tests, such as fetal scalp sampling (in which a tiny sample of the baby's blood is taken from its scalp and tested for oxygen content) may be used to confirm the diagnosis of fetal distress, especially if there is an element of doubt about the meaning of the heart rate tracing.

A lot of C-sections done for fetal distress are probably unnecessary. Many babies who experience even prolonged oxygen deprivation during labor probably will sustain no permanent brain damage. Unfortunately, it is very difficult to determine which babies are in danger of suffering irreparable damage. Obviously, no obstetrician wants to wait until the damage is done; at that point, the diagnosis is easy—but by then it's too late. Caesarean section should be performed while the baby is still healthy if fetal distress is strongly suspected. Yet when that healthy baby is delivered, it is often impossible to determine if the obstetrician acted too quickly, or acted prudently to avoid permanent injury.

In most situations, it is no longer considered necessary to have a repeat C-section if you had one in a previous delivery, provided that the incision made in the uterus was transverse—that is, made horizontally across the uterus. Vaginal birth after a previous C-section is commonly referred to by the acronym VBAC. Women have the option of requesting a repeat C-section, and many do, especially if they had a particularly difficult first labor. However, if you had a vertical incision on your uterus the first time, C-section will be recommended. Vertical incisions are considered less likely to withstand the stress and strain of contractions.

There are also some uncommon situations in which C-section is always necessary and appropriate. These include *placenta previa* (when the placenta blocks the cervix), heavy bleeding and *cord prolapse* (when the umbilical cord falls out before the baby is delivered). In these cases, C-section is undoubtedly a life-saving procedure.

What should you expect if you have a C-section? The first decision to be made, after the decision for the C-section itself, is the type of anesthesia to be used. If you already have an epidural catheter in place, extra medication can be given through the catheter to make you completely numb and pain-free below the chest. If you do not have an epidural, it is often quicker and easier to be given a spinal anesthetic. In both cases, you will have excellent pain relief and be awake and aware for the entire procedure. In the rare cases when minutes may mean the difference between life and death, general anesthesia will be used. In that case, you will be asleep for the duration of the surgery.

A nurse will put a catheter in your bladder, to continually drain out the urine. The bladder sits virtually of top of the uterus while the mother is lying on her back. If the bladder if full, it will be in the way during surgery. The nurse may also need to shave your pubic hair to clear the area where the incision will be made.

In the operating room, you will be placed on the operating table. Your arms will rest on boards on either side. The anesthesiologist will attach all sorts of monitoring devices that will be used to monitor your heart rate, blood pressure, and the oxygen content of your blood. You will, of course, already have an intravenous line in place to receive any fluids or medication you might need during the surgery. The procedures and the equipment may be intimidating, but they are all painless.

Your abdomen will be washed with a disinfectant soap, and the surgical drapes will be placed over your whole body, except your head. Then the surgery will begin, although you will not feel it. If you are awake, your labor coach can be with you and at your side, throughout the whole procedure.

A C-section usually takes 45 minutes to an hour to complete. It takes less than 10 minutes to get the baby out. The rest of the time is required to suture the incision in the uterus and abdominal wall. Repeat C-sections often take longer, however, because of the presence of scar tissue.

You will be able to see your baby immediately after it is born, and your coach can hold it, once it is cleaned and diapered. After the surgery is over, you will be transferred to the recovery room for several hours of observation. If you feel up to it, you can nurse the baby for the first time.

The recovery period for a C-section is longer than that for a vaginal delivery. You should expect to be in the hospital for three to four days, and you will most certainly need to take pain medication to ease the incisional pain.

There is no reason to feel disappointed if you have a C-section. After all, the object of pregnancy and labor is to deliver a healthy baby, and sometimes the only way to achieve that is by C-section.

Making the Incision

1 After the abdomen has been washed with disinfectant soap and the surgical drapes have been arranged, a scapel is used to make the initial incision into the skin of the abdomen. There are two types of skin incision that can be used. In this illustration, the *Pfannenstiel* or *transverse incision* is being created. Most C-sections are performed with this type of incision, also known as a *bikini cut*. The scar will not show even when you are lucky enough to be able to wear a bikini again. In emergency situations, a vertical incision (depicted by the dotted line), extending from the navel to slightly above the pubic bone, is used.

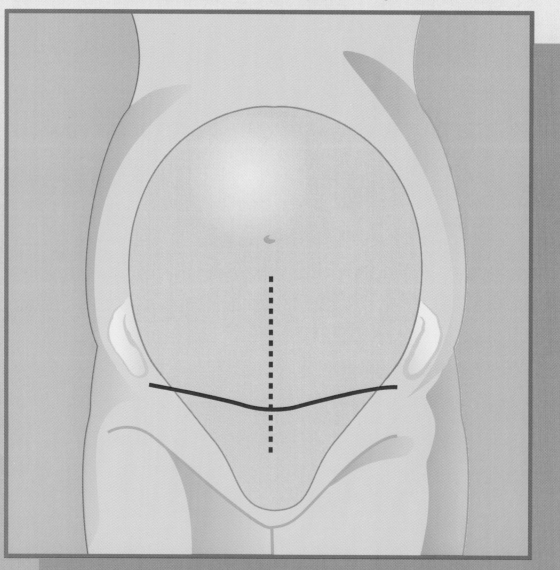

2 After the skin incision is created, multiple layers of tissue beneath the skin are carefully opened. Ultimately, the abdominal cavity is reached. The uterus is immediately visible, as it is the largest structure within the cavity. The bladder, which is located immediately in front of the uterus, is carefully pushed down from its usual location to prevent injury to it during the delivery of the baby.

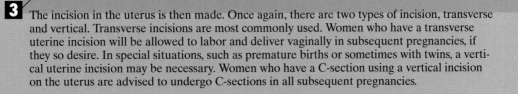

3 The incision in the uterus is then made. Once again, there are two types of incision, transverse and vertical. Transverse incisions are most commonly used. Women who have a transverse uterine incision will be allowed to labor and deliver vaginally in subsequent pregnancies, if they so desire. In special situations, such as premature births or sometimes with twins, a vertical uterine incision may be necessary. Women who have a C-section using a vertical incision on the uterus are advised to undergo C-sections in all subsequent pregnancies.

Delivery of the Baby and Closing of the Uterus

2 Once the presenting part has been delivered, the surgical assistant pushes on the mother's upper abdomen to force the rest of the baby out of the uterus under the guidance of the obstetrician. This is the only part of the operation that the mother is likely to feel. That's because epidural and spinal anesthesia can take away sensations of pain, but not sensations of pressure. Once the umbilical cord is clamped and cut, the baby is handled to the waiting nurse or pediatrician.

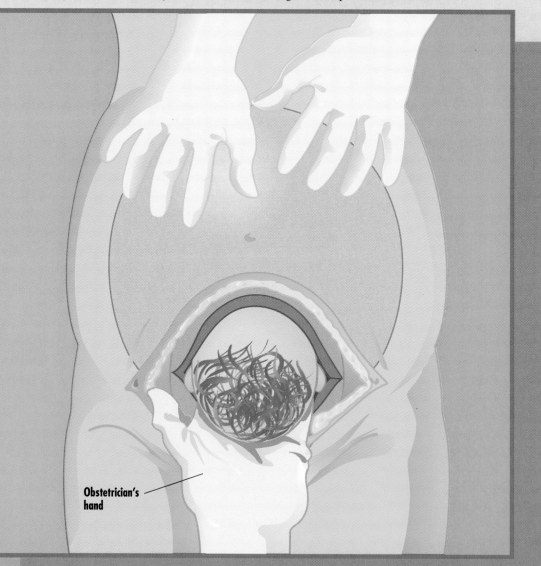

Obstetrician's hand

1 After the uterus has been opened, the obstetrician reaches into the lower part of the uterus, maneuvering his or her hand to cup the presenting (lowermost) part of the baby. In the case of a baby that was presenting head first, this will be the head. In breech presentations, this part will be the breech. The baby's presenting part is then lifted out of the pelvis and through the incision. A fair amount of effort by the obstetrician is sometimes required, especially if the head has descended deep into the pelvis before the surgery was begun.

3 After the placenta is removed from the uterus, the uterine incision is closed with surgical sutures. The initial closure is reinforced with a second layer of sutures. Then, the rest of the procedure is completed by closing each layer of the abdomen in the reverse order in which it was opened. The skin incision is usually closed with surgical staples, which look like paper staples, but are much easier to remove. A dressing is then applied to the skin incision and the surgery is completed.

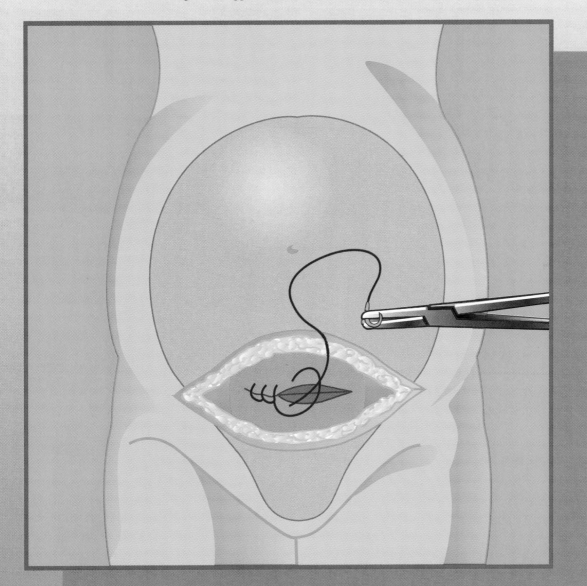

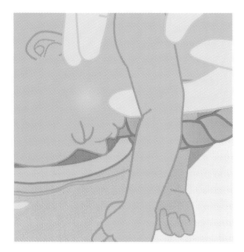

Breech Babies: Version and Delivery Techniques

APPROXIMATELY 4% OF BABIES will enter the last month of gestation in the breech presentation. When the baby is in the breech position, the obstetrician may attempt to turn it to the head down position. This turning is known as *version*.

The idea behind version is quite simple. The obstetrician attempts to manipulate the baby to shift into a more favorable position. Usually that means encouraging the baby to perform a forward somersault, changing direction 180 degrees. If the version succeeds, the head will become the presenting part, and vaginal delivery will be much more likely and safer.

Unfortunately, version is not appropriate in all situations and is not without risks. It is appropriate only in a single pregnancy where the position of the baby can be accurately diagnosed (usually by ultrasound). It is not appropriate for multiple pregnancies. The baby should not be unusually large and the presenting part should not be deep in the pelvis. Also, there must be a normal amount of amniotic fluid. All these conditions ensure that the baby has room to turn and will not be injured by the manipulations of the obstetrician's hands. In addition, a non-stress test must be reactive (indicating fetal well-being), and there should be no signs of placental problems (for example, low fluid, growth retardation, or vaginal bleeding). Version may represent a stress to the baby, and if there is evidence that the baby is not receiving adequate oxygen and nutrients at rest, it should not be attempted.

Version must be performed at the hospital because of the small but significant chance of causing fetal distress by turning the baby. If the baby experiences slowing of the heart rate after turning (bradycardia), perhaps because of the umbilical cord tangling, emergency C-section delivery will be required.

The actual procedure is quite simple. The mother reclines on a firm table. An ultrasound, to confirm fetal position, and a non-stress test, to demonstrate fetal well-being, are done. Some obstetricians will administer a dose of terbutaline by injection before the procedure to prevent uterine contractions. The mother's abdomen is dusted with powder to allow the obstetrician's hands to slide across it easily. The obstetrician uses one hand to pull the presenting part up out of the pelvis. With the first hand cupping the presenting part, the obstretician's other hand is placed at the back of the baby's head. Both hands are used to induce the baby to do a forward somersault. If the attempt succeeds, gentle pressure is exerted to push the head into the pelvis. The fetal heart rate should be monitored again to make sure that the new position does not cause fetal distress.

Version is successful approximately half the time. Not every baby will turn, and some babies who turn easily will turn back to their original position shortly after the procedure is completed. Nonetheless, if your obstetrician is comfortable and experienced with the procedure and there are no problems indicated, version is often worth trying. If successful, version reduces the risk to the baby from breech vaginal delivery, and the risk to the mother from C-section delivery.

Although the risks associated with vaginal delivery from the breech presentation are much higher than the risk of delivery head first, many breech babies do well when delivered vaginally. In recent years, there has been a small but growing number of women who have decided to forego C-section and attempt vaginal delivery. Years of experience before C-sections became routine helped to identify those types of breech positions that are at highest risk. This information can help parents make a more informed decision.

There are three types of breech presentation. The difference among the types is the position of the baby's legs relative to the rest of the body. *Frank breech*, in which the baby's legs are folded up against its body, is the most common type. The entire breech usually fills the pelvis and the baby's relatively compact position makes a vaginal delivery more likely. The frank breech presentation is the safest for vaginal delivery.

Even if the baby is in the frank breech presentation, however, there are a number of other criteria it should meet before proceeding with a vaginal delivery. Ultrasound examination should show that the baby is not unusually large and that the head is *flexed* (tilted forward). Entrapment of the head is more likely for babies who are unusually large or whose heads are not flexed.

If the decision is made to attempt breech vaginal delivery, close monitoring and careful observation of the progress of labor is mandatory. Any indication that the baby is too large to fit, such as slow progress in labor, should be regarded as a signal that C-section is the safer course. This is because the body is smaller than the head. If the body is having difficulty fitting through the pelvis, the head will never fit, especially because there is no time for it to undergo molding, as it would if it were passing through the pelvis head first.

If labor progresses smoothly, successful vaginal delivery is more likely. As in normal labor, the cervix dilates to 10 cm. Then the breech baby must be pushed out.

In the frank breech presentation, the buttocks are born first. The body is allowed to slide out with the obstetrician's support. After the abdomen is out, the obstetrician gently rotates the baby to either side, in preparation for delivery of the arms. This ensures that the arms are free and not accidentally trapped behind the baby's head. After the arms are born, the shoulders follow.

Now it is time for the head to be born. The delivery of the head can be assisted by a variety of maneuvers, all of which attempt to keep the head flexed as it is gently delivered. This is the most critical part of the delivery, because the possibility always remains that the head could become trapped behind the pubic bone. In difficult cases, special forceps may be required to deliver the head. Once the head has been delivered, everyone breathes a big sigh of relief. The cord is clamped and cut and the baby is thoroughly examined to make sure that no injuries have occurred.

Other breech presentations are not considered safe to attempt vaginal delivery. In the *complete breech*, the baby looks as if it is sitting Indian style, with its legs crossed in front of it. As you might imagine, it is difficult, if not impossible, for the baby to pass through the pelvis in this position.

A *footling breech* has one leg (single footling breech) or both legs (double footling breech) underneath it. The feet lead the way in passing through the pelvis. Although the feet fit easily, their small size creates another problem. As the cervix dilates, the umbilical cord may fall down around the baby's feet. When the membranes rupture, the cord may fall out of the uterus altogether (this is known as *cord prolapse*). This is an emergency. When the cord falls out of the warm, wet environment of the uterus into the vagina it may go into spasm, completely cutting off the flow of blood and depriving the baby of oxygen. Emergency C-section is required to deliver the baby as soon as possible. Cord prolapse is a fairly common complication of labor in single or double footling breech babies.

Women contemplating vaginal breech delivery are advised that only the frank breech presentation is safe. The complete breech or the footling breech should be delivered by C-section. It is important to remember, however, that even if the baby is in the frank breech presentation, and all the other criteria for vaginal delivery are met, there is still a significantly higher risk of injury to the baby by vaginal delivery than by head-first delivery or by C-section.

Breech Presentations

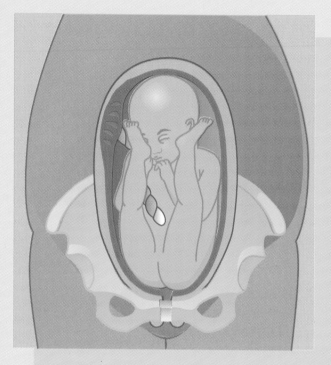

Frank breech   This is the most common type of breech presentation and the safest for vaginal delivery. The legs are folded against the baby's body, and the relatively compact size makes it fairly easy for the baby to pass through the pelvis. The breech fills the pelvis until it is delivered, which makes it much less likely that the umbilical cord can prolapse through the cervix.

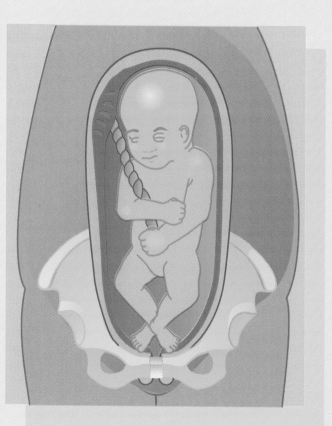

Double footling breech   The baby's legs are underneath it. When labor begins, the legs will descend first. Notice that this position leaves room for the umbilical cord to fall down to the level of the cervix. After the membranes rupture, the cord may fall out through the open cervix, go into spasm, and cut off the baby's oxygen supply. Cord prolapse is an obstetric emergency requiring immediate delivery.

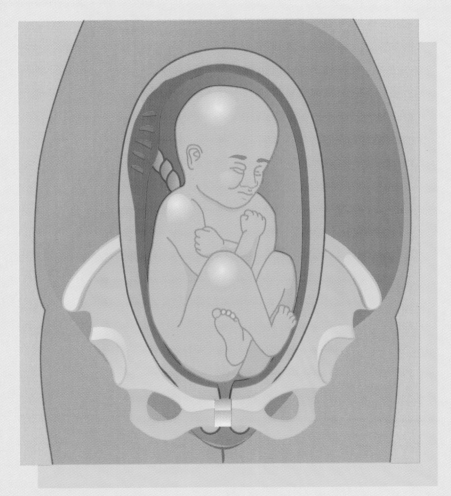

Complete breech   The baby appears to be sitting, with legs crossed, in the pelvis. This position of the legs makes it nearly impossible for the baby to pass through the pelvis, and vaginal delivery is not considered safe.

The Mother During Version

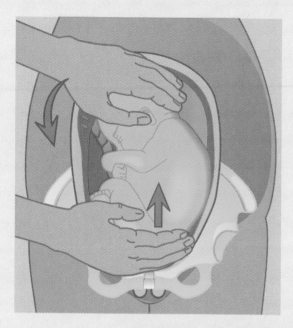

Notice that the obstetrician's hands are positioned to lift the breech out of the pelvis and encourage the baby to do a forward somersault. You can see that a large baby or a baby positioned deep in the pelvis will be unable to turn. Care must be taken to avoid disturbing the placenta. The baby should be monitored carefully after version to make sure that it is not stressed by the new position.

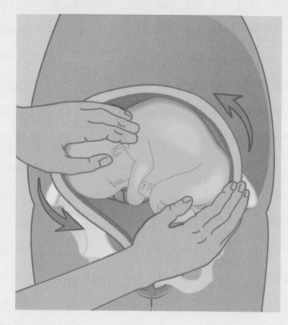

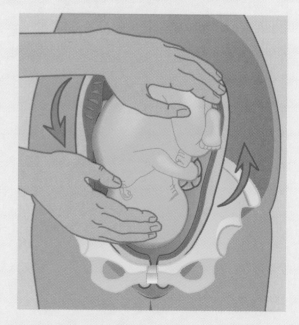

Delivery of the After-Coming Head

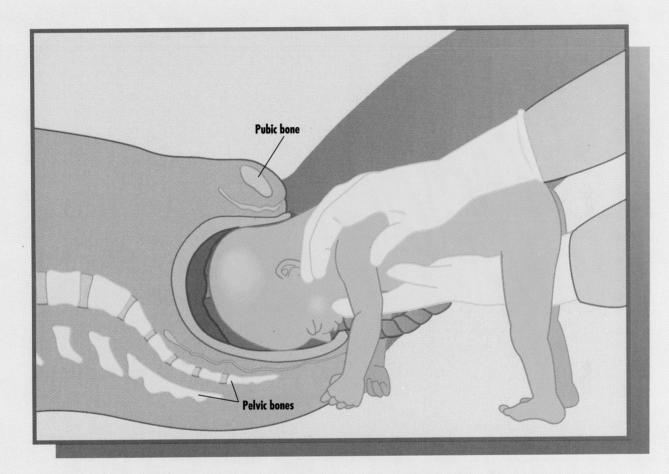

The baby's body has been delivered easily, but the most critical part of the delivery is still to come. Notice the close relationship between the baby's head and the mother's pelvic bones. The baby's head is its biggest part, and it may become trapped, even if the baby's body had no difficulty negotiating the pelvis. In many cases, the baby's head can be delivered easily. There are a variety of maneuvers available, including special forceps, to complete the delivery of the head, if difficulty is encountered. However, if the head does not deliver easily, the chance of injury to the head or neck is high. Time is of the essence in delivering the after-coming head. As you can see, the umbilical cord is outside the mother's body. It is most likely in spasm now, preventing oxygen transfer from the placenta to the baby. In addition, the baby's mouth and nose are still inside the vagina, making it impossible for the baby to draw a breath.

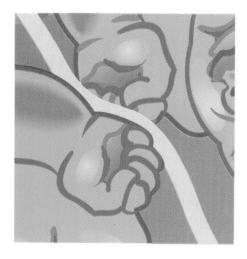

How Twins Are Delivered

HAVING TWINS MORE than doubles the trial and tribulation of a single pregnancy and delivery. That's because there are a variety of complaints and risks that are much more common in twin pregnancies than in single ones, and there are new conditions that do not arise at all in singleton pregnancies.

There are two types of twins, fraternal and identical. Fraternal twins result from two separate ova fertilized by two different sperm. Although they share nine months together in the uterus, fraternal twins are no more closely related genetically than any other siblings. Identical twins occur when one already fertilized ovum splits into two equal parts. Each baby that subsequently develops is genetically identical to the other. That's why identical twins are always of the same sex and look very much alike.

Initially, twin pregnancies develop just like singleton pregnancies. There is more than enough room in the uterus for two embryos to grow without crowding. The only early symptom of a twin pregnancy may be increased morning sickness, probably due to a higher level of pregnancy-related hormones. The mother's first clue of a developing twin pregnancy, however, may be a larger-than-expected uterus at her first prenatal exam.

The best tool for accurately diagnosing twin pregnancy is ultrasound. Each embryo or fetus is plainly visible, usually within its own amniotic sac. If twins are not diagnosed in early pregnancy, later signs that may arouse suspicion include a uterine size consistently larger than gestational age would indicate, and two distinct fetal heart rates. These signs can be detected by a test called a Doppler exam.

As the pregnancy progresses, uterine crowding does occurs. Before 20 weeks of gestation, each twin is usually the same size as a singleton fetus of equivalent age. After 20 weeks, each twin tends to grow more slowly. That's why twins, even if not premature, tend to have a lower than average birth weight.

The most common problem associated with twin pregnancy is a much higher risk of premature labor. The absolute size of the babies does not seem to be the source of the problem. After all, 28-week twins weigh much less than a single fetus at term. The higher risk of premature labor seems to be related to the rapid rate of change in uterine size. Most practitioners will recommend more frequent prenatal visits for twin pregnancies because of the increased risk of premature labor and pre-eclampsia. Starting at 26 weeks, or the end of the second trimester, the obstetrician or midwife will usually perform a cervical exam at each visit to check for early dilatation of the cervix. When the third trimester begins, many practitioners recommend that the mother decrease her normal activity level, often suggesting cutting back on work and instituting a period of bed rest each day.

The well-being of a singleton fetus is generally assessed by measuring fundal height, which should correspond to gestational age (for an explanation of fundal height, see Chapter 4). In twin pregnancies, there is no correspondence between fundal height and gestational age. Moreover, even if the fundal height is greater at each prenatal visit than at the preceding one, there is no way of knowing whether both babies are growing equally. That's why, starting at 32 weeks, routine ultrasound evaluations are recommended every two weeks. Non-stress testing is also performed every two weeks. This monitoring can detect subtle signs that each placenta is not meeting the needs of the baby, which is much more common in twin pregnancies.

The delivery of twins also presents the possiblity of many more combinations of fetal positions than singleton deliveries. The first twin may be head first in the pelvis (vertex), but the second twin may be vertex, breech, or transverse. In fact, each twin is much less likely to present in the vertex position than is a singleton fetus.

Planning for delivery usually starts with consideration of the position of the first (presenting) twin. If the presenting twin is breech or transverse, C-section is recommended, particularly if (as is often the case) the twins are premature. Breech delivery is much riskier for a premature baby because the ratio of head size to body size is much greater than for full-term babies. The premature baby's body will always slip out easily, but the head is more likely to become trapped.

If the first twin is in the vertex position, plans are usually made to attempt vaginal delivery. Even if the second twin is breech or transverse, it often changes position once its sibling has been born. Additionally, version can be attempted after the delivery of the first twin. The second twin is often smaller and has plenty of room to turn once the first twin has been born. Of course, the second twin may not cooperate, and the decision must be made at that time whether to deliver it from the breech presentation or to perform a C-section. This can only be determined by consideration of the situation at hand; no general rules apply.

Twins must be monitored very carefully in labor, and there are special monitors designed for just this purpose. The monitors can record two heart rate patterns in addition to recording the contraction pattern. It is possible for one fetus to develop signs of distress during labor while the other appears to tolerate labor well. Decisions about whether to intervene will always be based on the condition of the baby that is doing poorly, even if its sibling is fine.

After the first twin is delivered, the second twin is at risk of *placental abruption*. In this condition, the placenta begins to separate from the wall of the uterus before the baby is born. Placental abruption can happen in singleton pregnancies, but it is rare. It is more common in twin pregnancies after the first twin is born because the uterus has already begun to shrink in size, initiating the normal process of placental detachment. If placental abruption occurs after the delivery of the first twin, emergency C-section may be required, even if the second twin is in the vertex (head first) presentation. That's because no fetus can tolerate the decreased oxygen supply that accompanies significant placental separation.

The Development and Positioning of Twins

Fraternal twins develop from two separate ova fertilized by two different sperm. Fraternal twins are no more closely related genetically than other siblings, even though they share nine months together in the uterus.

Identical twins result when a fertilized ovum splits into two equal parts. Each baby that subsequently develops is genetically identical to the other. That's why identical twins are always of the same sex and look very much alike.

Vertex-vertex twins This is the most favorable position for successful vaginal delivery. The first twin will be born head first. The second twin is likely to descend head first into the pelvis after its sibling has been born. There is, of course, no guarantee that the second twin will cooperate; there will be enough room available for the second twin to change position after the first twin is delivered, but this is rare.

Vertex-breech twins   Many sets of twins favor this position. The first twin will be delivered head first. The second is likely to descend in the breech presentation unless an attempt is made to turn it by version. There is some controversy in obstetrical practice about how to handle a second twin that does not turn. Some practitioners are willing to deliver the second baby from the breech presentation, reasoning that a baby's head has just passed through the pelvis successfully, even though it is not the head of the baby in question, but that of its sibling. Other practitioners may recommend a C-section, particularly if the second twin is much larger than the first. The same management plan applies to twins in the vertex-transverse position. The only difference is that if the second twin descends in the transverse position, C-section is a definite necessity.

Breech-vertex twins   The method of delivery of twins in this position is dictated by the presentation of the first twin. As in the case of a single fetus in the breech position, C-section is usually recommended. Similarly, if the first twin is in the transverse position, C-section will be required, because a baby in the transverse position is undeliverable vaginally.

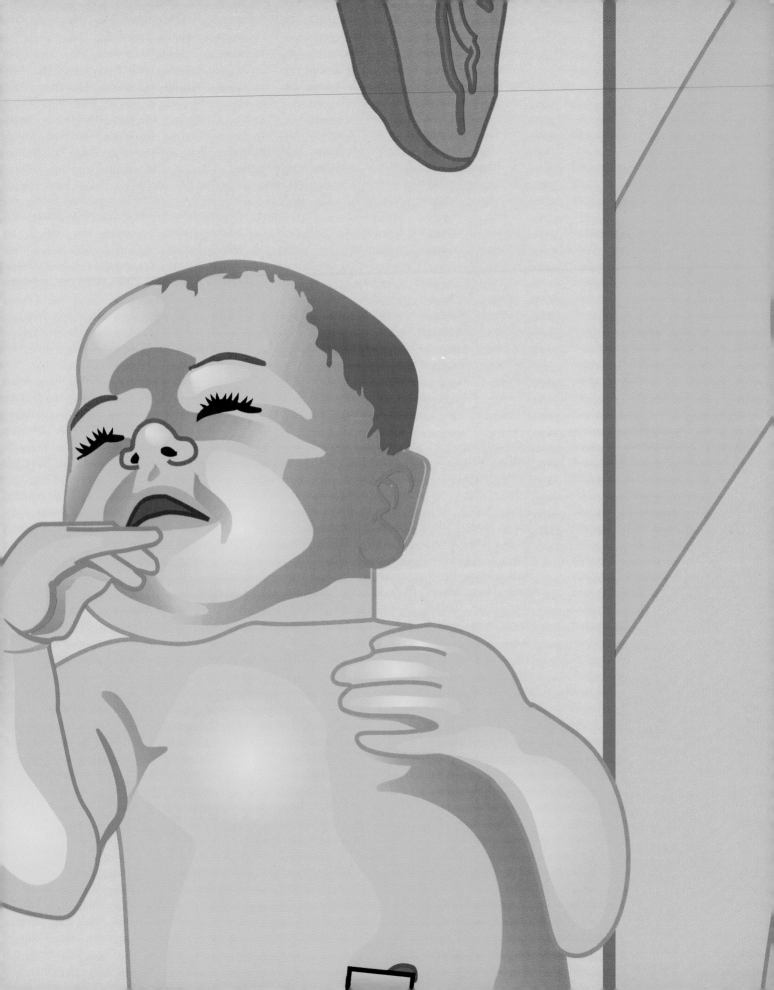

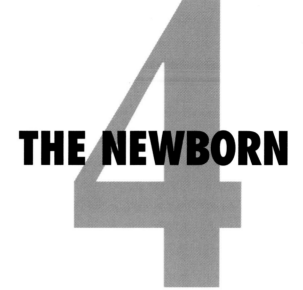

THE NEWBORN

LABOR MAY TAKE many paths and delivery may occur in many ways, but there is one thing common to all deliveries. After the practitioner's cry of "It's a boy" or "It's a girl," every parent asks the same question: "Is my baby okay?" Most parents first concern is whether all the body parts are present and accounted for. "Are there ten finger and ten toes?" is usually the parents' second question. But obstetricians, midwives, and pediatricians are concerned not just about body parts, but whether the baby can make the virtually instantaneous transformation from being supported by the placenta to surviving on its own.

During the first few minutes after birth, miraculous changes take place in the baby's body. The lungs, which are partially collapsed when the baby is in the uterus, must expand and begin to absorb oxygen. The circulation must change from one that includes and is dependent upon the placenta to the normal circulation, which is self-supporting. These changes, described in Chapter 28, are often virtually completed within the time it takes for the baby to draw its first few breaths and give a lusty wail.

There are a variety of factors that obstetricians and pediatricians take into account when evaluating the newborn's efforts to adjust to life outside the uterus. Each factor can be scored with points, and the total score gives a fairly good approximation of how well the baby is doing. This scoring system is known as the Apgar score, and it is discussed in detail in Chapter 29.

Although the newborn's ability to meet its oxygen requirements shifts from dependence on the mother to self-sufficiency, there is little else that it can do for itself. Indeed, it is designed to continue receiving all nutrition from its mother in the form of breast milk. Breast-feeding provides the perfect food for the newborn. Colostrum, which is secreted in the hours immediately following delivery, transmits important antibodies to the baby, providing additional protection from the common diseases of early childhood. Breast milk itself is always available, always the right temperature, and always present in the perfect quantity.

Although breast-feeding is a natural function, neither a new mother nor a brand-new baby knows exactly how to begin. The art of breast-feeding must be learned through trial and error; but with a bit of patience on the mother's part (babies are never patient), this skill can usually be mastered in a few days. Chapter 30 details the process of breast-feeding and the necessary steps to begin the nursing partnership.

Regardless of whether you breast-feed or bottle-feed, your newborn baby is dependent on you for love and care. The end of pregnancy represents a new beginning, filled with new joys and fears and new excitements and responsibilities.

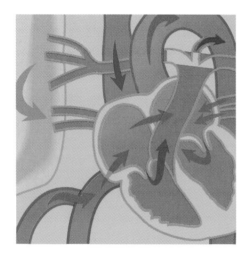

How Your Baby Begins to Breathe

WHILE THE BABY is being born, everyone's eyes are focused on the star as the grand entrance is accomplished. But the spectators are waiting not just for the appearance of the baby; its first sounds are also eagerly anticipated. A loud and lusty cry is the proof that the baby has made the transition to its new environment safely and can now breathe on its own.

In order to understand the miraculous changes that take place in the first few moments after birth, it is necessary to examine the way the fetal blood circulation works. There are two critical differences between fetal circulation and newborn circulation. The first difference is that oxygen is delivered to the fetus across the placenta and into the umbilical cord. This oxygenated blood is returned to the fetus's heart and then pumped out to the rest of the body. The second difference is that the fetal lungs do not serve a function and, therefore, receive only a small fraction of the circulation as compared to the circulation requirements after birth.

These important differences are reflected in structural differences within the heart itself during the course of gestation. Although the fetal heart contains the same four chambers and blood vessels that the child or adult heart contains, the chambers and blood vessels relate to each other in different ways. For example, the two upper chambers of the heart, the left and right *atria*, are open to each other through a special passage (the *foramen ovale*) during gestation. Additionally, although a large amount of blood is pumped out to the lungs through the pulmonary artery, a lot of it is diverted to the main circulation by way of a special channel (the *ductus arteriosus*) before it gets to the lungs. These structural differences ensure that very little oxygen is wasted by pumping it through the fetal lungs, which are virtually useless and, in fact, are partially collapsed within the chest.

This all changes in the first few moments after birth. Probably a variety of stimuli contribute to the newborn's tremendous urge to inhale its first lungful of air. These stimuli include the rapidly falling oxygen concentration and rapidly rising carbon dioxide concentration as the umbilical vessels constrict. The compression of the fetal chest in the birth canal and its sudden release also may contribute to the urge to breathe.

When the newborn draws its first breath, its lungs expand to almost full capacity; at this point, the relationships among the organs in the chest change dramatically. The lungs, which previously could accept only a small amount of the blood leaving the heart, now can accept much more. Not only can they accept more blood flow, it is imperative that they receive it, because this is the new source of oxygen.

This dramatic shift in the amount of blood flow changes the blood pressure within each chamber of the heart. As the pressure rises in the left atrium, a flap of tissue is pushed over the foramen ovale, effectively closing this passage between the two atria. Additionally, the ductus arteriosus, the channel that previously drained blood away from the lungs, constricts, ensuring that all the blood pumped out to the lungs actually reaches the lungs. There, the blood will pick up its load of oxygen, before returning to the heart to be pumped out to the rest of the body.

The blood vessels of the umbilical cord are instantly rendered obsolete. If they have not constricted already, they will do so after the baby takes its first few breaths. This process is aided by the clamping of the umbilical cord. The umbilical vessels will atrophy and the remnant of the umbilical cord still attached to the baby will dry up and fall off. The place where the umbilical cord was attached to the baby will forever be marked by the navel, also known as the *umbilicus*.

These amazing changes take place within moments after birth. The baby's first cry is not a cry of protest, but a cry of life, announcing that the transition between the uterus and the outside world has been safely negotiated. For this reason, the newborn's first cry is music to the ears of obstetricians, midwives, and new parents.

The Fetal Circulation

4 Some of the blood flow does pass from the right atrium to the right ventricle and out toward the lungs. A significant portion of this flow is diverted into the main circulation by way of a special channel, the *ductus arteriosus*. This is another measure that increases circulation efficiency. Only a minimal amount of oxygenated blood ever reaches the lungs. Most of the oxygenated blood is pumped out to the rest of the body's organs, where it is needed to sustain life and growth.

3 In the fetus, the right and left *atria* are open to each other through a special passage, the *foramen ovale*. This passage allows blood to travel across the heart, bypassing the lungs. In the fetus whose lungs serve virtually no purpose, this is a more efficient mode of circulation.

2 The umbilical vein carries the oxygenated blood from the placenta to the heart. The heart pumps the oxygenated blood out to the rest of the body.

1 The fetus receives its oxygen supply from the placenta.

The Newborn Circulation

3 When the lungs expand, they are capable of accepting a much larger amount of blood flow than they could before birth. This changes the blood pressure within each chamber of the heart and the blood pressure relationships between the four chambers. As the pressure rises in the left atrium, a flap of tissue is pushed over the foramen ovale, thereby closing the passage between the two atria. All of the blood flow that formerly crossed the foramen ovale and was diverted away from the lungs is now pumped out directly to the lungs instead.

4 The *ductus arteriosus* constricts immediately after birth, probably in response to the rising concentration of oxygen in the blood which is flowing through it. This effectively closes the other path that diverted blood flow away from the lungs. Now, all the blood leaving the heart proceeds first to the lungs to pick up oxygen, then returns to the left side of the heart, then is pumped out again to supply the oxygen needs of the rest of the body.

2 Now the lungs are the only source of oxygen. It is critical that they receive a large portion of the blood flow from every beat of the heart. The oxygenated blood is returned to the left side of the heart and then pumped out again to the rest of the body.

1 At the moment of birth the placenta becomes obsolete. It is imperative that the massive amount of blood flow to and from the placenta be reduced immediately. This occurs when the umbilical vessels constrict in response to contact with the cooler temperature of the air. This process is aided by clamping and cutting the umbilical cord.

Clamp

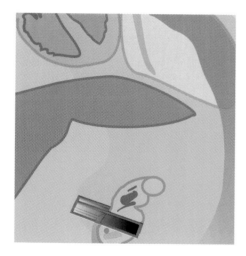

How the Newborn is Evaluated

I T'S EASY TO tell that a newborn who has a loud and lusty cry, vigorously moves his or her arms and legs, and protests mightily when disturbed has made an excellent transition to the outside world. Conversely, no special medical training is needed to understand that a newborn who makes no attempt to breathe, is listless and does not react to stimulation, requires immediate medical attention to assist in adjusting to the environment outside of the womb. However, between these two extremes, there is a broad spectrum of possible responses that a newborn can exhibit, and a precise way of evaluating the infant's critical physiological adjustment process was clearly needed.

In 1952, Dr. Virginia Apgar, an anesthesiologist, met that need by developing a system to evaluate newborn response within the first five minutes after birth. Five different characteristics are observed and scored. The total number of points is referred to as the Apgar score. More than 40 years after it was introduced, this scoring system remains a vital tool in assessing the newborn infant.

It is very important to keep in mind that Apgar scores are *not* measures of intelligence or brain function. They are merely a shorthand way of conveying information about the newborn's initial adjustment to the outside world. Apgar scores have virtually no prognostic significance. This means that they cannot predict an infant's future health, intelligence, or anything else.

The Apgar scoring system evaluates five different characteristics of the newborn: heart rate, respiratory effort, muscle tone, reflex irritability, and color. Each characteristic can be rated from 0 to 2, with 0 as the worst score and 2 as the best. The total number of points is the Apgar score itself. The highest possible score is 10, although even the healthiest newborns are rarely rated 10. Usually, that's because of the color score. It can take many hours for a newborn to become a healthy color all the way down to the fingertips and toes.

The Apgar score is calculated twice: first at 1 minute and then at 5 minutes. The 1-minute Apgar score indicates whether a newborn requires help in making the all-important transition to breathing on its own. If a newborn has a low 1-minute Apgar score, he or she will probably receive assistance such as stimulation by rubbing with a warm blanket (the slap on the bottom is found only in old movies), supplemental oxygen, and suctioning of the mouth and nose to remove residual amniotic fluid. If the infant does not respond to these measures, a pediatrician may pass a tiny breathing tube into the baby's lungs to pump oxygen in and out of the lungs until the baby can breathe independently.

Most infants respond promptly to such assistance. The 5-minute Apgar score reflects the baby's response to these measures. By 5 minutes after birth, most babies, even those with low 1-minute Apgar scores, will have a score of 8 or 9. At 5 minutes, if the baby still has a score that is lower than 7, further assistance will be necessary.

It can be extremely frightening to watch nurses and doctors working over your new baby, coaxing him or her to take those first few breaths. In this situation, 5 minutes can feel like 5 hours. Yet when you consider the miraculous transition that birth requires, it is not surprising that many babies need a little help at first. It helps you to know that within the first 5 minutes almost all babies begin to breathe on their own. You will be happy and relieved when you hear those angry cries, signaling to all present, "Leave me alone; I can do it by myself!"

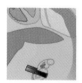

The Apgar Scoring System

The Apgar scoring system evaluates five different characteristics of the newborn: heart rate, respiratory effort, muscle tone, reflex irritability, and color. Each characteristic can be rated from 0 to 2, with 0 as the worst score and 2 as the best. The total number of points is the Apgar score itself. The highest possible score is 10, although even the healthiest newborns are rarely rated 10.

Heart rate   A normal newborn heart rate is much faster than that of an older child or adult. The newborn receives a score of 2 for a heart rate over 100 and a score of 1 for a heart rate under 100. A 0 is given if no heart rate can be detected. This is a sign that infant CPR should be initiated immediately.

Respiratory effort   The newborn should make vigorous attempts to initiate breathing. Strong, successful attempts will be reflected in a loud cry and that baby will receive a score of 2. If respiratory effort is weak or breathing is irregular, the baby will receive a score of 1. A score of 0 is given if the newborn makes no attempt to breathe, or if immediate assistance is required, either with an oxygen mask or a breathing tube.

Muscle tone   A newborn may receive a score of 2 for actively moving his or her limbs about. A score of 1 is given if the arms and legs are flexed but not moving. A score of 0 is reserved for babies who are limp. This is another sign that the newborn requires assistance in initiating breathing.

2 1 0

Reflex irritability   The process of birth itself is very stimulating, and the typical newborn will respond vigorously to additional stimulation. The practitioner may rub the baby's face or tap his or her feet in order to elicit a response. The baby receives a score of 2 for crying shortly after delivery. A score of 1 is given if the baby grimaces in response to stimulation. If the baby demonstrates no response to stimulation, a score of 0 is given.

Color   At the moment of birth, most babies are, surprisingly, a shade of blue. Within the first minute, however, the head and body turn to a color that indicates good oxygenation. If the entire body is a healthy color, the newborn will receive a score of 2. This is rare; most babies have blue hands and feet for several hours after birth. These babies receive a score of 1. A 0 is given if the baby remains blue, and assistance is required.

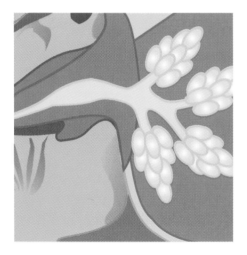

How Your Baby Begins Breast-Feeding

PREGNANCY CREATES A special relationship between mother and child. The baby rests safe and secure in the uterus, while its every need is easily met by the mother. After birth, the baby begins the long, slow process toward independence. Learning to absorb nutrition through the digestive tract rather than receiving nutrients through the umbilical cord is an important skill that must be perfected in the first few days after birth.

Nature has designed breast-feeding as the perfect system to ease this transition. The mother continues to process food into its nutrient components, but now these components are transported into the fluid produced by the breasts. Not only does breast milk contain all the necessary nutrients for the rapidly developing newborn, it has several other great advantages as well. Breast milk contains antibodies that pass the mother's immunity to common childhood illnesses directly to the baby; that's why breast-fed infants have fewer colds and ear infections than bottle-fed babies. Also, breast milk is always ready when the baby is hungry and is always the perfect temperature.

All these advantages incline most pregnant women to plan on breast-feeding. Nonetheless, only 56 percent of new mothers leave the hospital with plans to breast-feed exclusively. The statistics are even more disappointing three weeks after birth. In that time, many new mothers give up on nursing. However, of the remaining women who are still breast-feeding at three weeks, most will continue breast-feeding for six months, which is the length of time that breast milk offers its maximal beneficial effect.

Why do so many women have trouble initiating and maintaining breast-feeding if it is nature's intended method for nourishing infants? There are two main reasons for this phenomenon. The first is that many women, believing that breast-feeding is natural, fail to understand that it requires a period of learning and adjustment for both mother and newborn. When they encounter the early, minor difficulties associated with establishing the nursing relationship, they think that something is wrong and they quit. The second reason is that formula is so accessible, and there is tremendous societal pressure to use it. Today, most new parents have mothers who never breast-fed. A lot of these older women are suspicious of breast-feeding and instead of offering support to their daughters and daughters-in-law, they offer criticism in the guise of interested questions or advice, such as "How do you know she's getting enough?" and "Looks to me like he's still hungry."

These simple comments are easily addressed by a confident new mother, but a confident new mother is hard to find. The typical first-time mother, still reeling from the hormonal surges surrounding delivery, is very insecure in her relationship with her newborn. Yet she is consumed with love for this helpless creature, and any suggestion, no matter how innocent, that she is starving her child is enough to send her to the drugstore for formula at any time of the day or night.

The key, then, to establishing and maintaining a satisfying breast-feeding relationship is knowledge. It is very important to understand how a baby *learns* to nurse. It is equally critical to understand how breast milk production is influenced.

The most important thing to remember about getting started breast-feeding is that it takes babies a while to figure out the mechanics of this practice. At first, they have no idea that they are eating until the milk begins to fill their stomach. This means that your baby does not recognize either the breast or the nipple. An infant does not understand that the nipple is the source of the milk. A baby does not even realize that the nipple is in its mouth unless certain parts of the mouth are stimulated. Only then will he or she *latch-on* and begin to suck. In a few days, the infant begins to make simple connections and learns to breast-feed. Until then, he or she is very easily frustrated and may have some difficulty getting started.

After all, babies only decide that they want to eat when they are very hungry. In just a few moments they become frantic with hunger. Being held next to the breast with the nipple near their mouth does nothing to soothe them. The nipple must be introduced into the mouth and stroked along the palate. Only then will the innate urge to suck be activated. The baby will latch-on to the nipple, the milk will begin to flow, and the baby who was frantic only moments before now relaxes completely, blissfully enjoying the sweet taste of the soothing liquid.

Breast-feeding operates under a feedback mechanism mediated by hormones. When the baby latches-on and begins to suck, the hormone *prolactin* is released from the pituitary gland. Prolactin stimulates the breasts to produce milk. That's why more breast-feeding produces more milk. Whatever the baby takes during one feeding will be replaced in time for the next feeding. In the beginning, the baby will want to nurse frequently, probably every two hours. The breasts build up the milk supply from zero to

1–2 ounces. After several days, once the milk supply has been established, the baby will receive more milk at each nursing session and be able to last longer between feedings.

The feedback mechanism has important consequences when a bottle of formula is substituted for a nursing session. Your body does not know that the baby received a bottle. It senses that the baby did not need to eat for a longer time than usual, and it cuts back on the milk available for the next nursing session. Your decreased milk supply leaves the baby hungry at the next nursing, prompting you to offer another bottle, thus setting up a vicious cycle. It does not take many days before you are tempted to give up nursing entirely because there was "not enough milk." It is important to remember that there is no such thing as not enough milk. Your milk supply will drop off only if you interfere with milk production by substituting bottles of formula for nursing. Many new mothers inadvertently sabotage their breast-feeding efforts in this way.

In addition, if you abruptly change the nursing schedule, your breasts will become engorged, that is, painfully full of milk. *Engorgement* is very uncomfortable and can lead to breast infection. If you wish to change the nursing schedule, there are several points to keep in mind. Never skip more than one feeding at a time. Never discontinue nursing abruptly. Always make changes over a period of days, so that your milk supply will decrease gradually. If you need to be away from the baby for a period of time, use a breast pump while you are gone. The milk you pump from your breast can be saved to bottle-feed the baby at another time and you will avoid engorgement.

Breast-feeding is not necessarily difficult or inconvenient. After all, until the relatively recent invention of formula, all babies were successfully breast-fed. If you plan on breast-feeding, learn all you can about the process. Be patient for the first few days while your baby learns to nurse. Above all, give yourself time. If you stick with breast-feeding for just two to three weeks, you may find that you enjoy it so much that many weeks or months of a delightful nursing relationship will surely follow.

Breast-Feeding

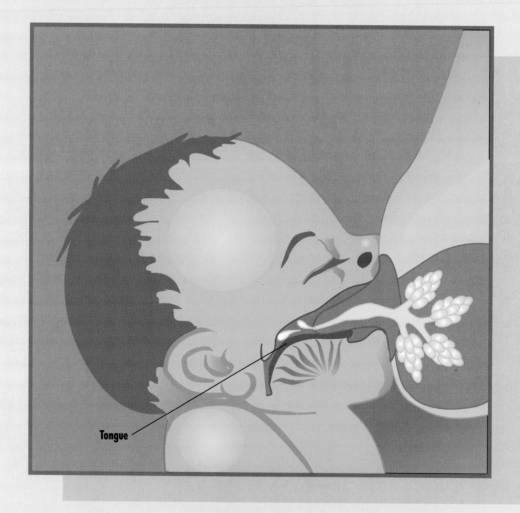

Tongue

1 To begin nursing, the baby must take the entire nipple and as much of the areola as possible into its mouth. This is known as latching-on. Although the milk comes out of the nipple, it is not released until the baby's tongue strokes the large milk ducts in the areola.

4 As the baby latches on, stimulation of the nipple and areola causes the hormone oxytocin to be released from the pituitary gland. This is the same hormone that causes contractions of the uterus during labor. Oxytocin causes similar contractions in the tiny glands of the breast, forcing milk out of the glands and toward the nipple. This is known as *let-down*. Oxytocin can still cause uterine contractions; that's why many women experience uterine cramping during the first few days of nursing. Breast-feeding actually stimulates the uterus to return to its pre-pregnancy size. The hormone prolactin is also released from the pituitary gland during breast-feeding. This hormone stimulates the breasts to produce more milk. The glands of the breast do not produce milk continuously; they produce milk in response to the emptying of the breasts and the production of prolactin when the baby sucks.

2 Proper nursing position is important to ensure that both mother and baby are comfortable. Although there are a variety of ways to hold the baby while nursing, the baby should always face the breast directly. This makes it much easier for the baby to latch-on and reduces painful pressure and pulling on the nipple.

Oxytocin and prolactin

3 In the first few days after birth, the baby receives colostrum from the breast. This "pre-milk" is very rich in antibodies, allowing the mother to pass on her immunities to various childhood illnesses to her baby. Only a small volume of colostrum is produced, but the baby does not become dehydrated because it is born with extra "water-weight" to sustain it for the first 48 hours. Emptying the breast of colostrum or milk stimulates the breast glands to produce more milk. This is part of the feedback mechanism that regulates breast-feeding. The more the baby nurses, the more milk is produced to replace it in time for the next feeding. As the baby nurses frequently during the first few days after delivery, the milk supply gradually increases. More milk becomes available at each feeding, which allows the baby to last longer between feedings.

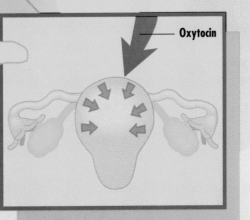

Oxytocin

transition of labor from active phase to
delivery, 98

transverse lie position, 74, 77

tubal (ectopic) pregnancy, 46

twins, 187–191

adjusting AFP results for, 36

U

ultrasound

checking for twins, 187, 188

checking growth of fetus, 15, 19, 48

described, 19, 21–22, 26–27

as diganostic tool, 3

to investigate causes of bleeding, 45, 48

for sex determination, 9

umbilical cord, 13, 74, 112, 122

considerations for version of breech babies,
179

cord prolapse, 171, 181, 182

obsolesence at birth, 198

umbilicus, 198

urinary tract infections, as cause of premature
labor, 51, 54

urination, increased urge for, 6

urine

fetal replacement after amniocentesis, 42

fetal waste discharges, 13

tests of mother's, 29, 30, 51

uterus. *See also* cervix; contractions; placenta

active and passive segments of, 85, 88

and cephalopelvic disproportion (CDP), 169

in first trimester, 6–7

and postpartum uterine bleeding, 106,
114–115

return to normal size, 19, 106

size and growth rate with twins, 187, 188

in third trimester, 19

uterine walls, 7

and vaginal birth after C-section, 171

V

vacuum extraction delivery, 153–154, 156–157

VBAC (vaginal birth after C-section), 171, 175

vernix, 13

version (fetal positioning prior to delivery),
74, 179–180, 184

of twins, 191

vertex, left occiput anterior position, 73

vertex, occiput posterior position, 73

vision problems, blurriness and high blood
pressure, 61

W

weight gain

by fetus, 18

by mothers, 5, 29, 32

of twins, 187

Ziff-Davis Press Survey of Readers

Please help us in our effort to produce the best books on personal computing.
For your assistance, we would be pleased to send you a FREE catalog
featuring the complete line of Ziff-Davis Press books.

1. How did you first learn about this book?

Recommended by a friend . . . . □ -1 (5)

Recommended by store personnel . . . . □ -2

Saw in Ziff-Davis Press catalog . . . . □ -3

Received advertisement in the mail . . . . □ -4

Saw the book on bookshelf at store . . . . □ -5

Read book review in: _____ □ -6

Saw an advertisement in: _____ □ -7

Other (Please specify): _____ □ -8

2. Which THREE of the following factors most influenced your decision to purchase this book? (Please check up to THREE.)

Front or back cover information on book . . . □ -1 (6)

Logo of magazine affiliated with book . . . . . . □ -2

Special approach to the content . . . . □ -3

Completeness of content . . . . □ -4

Author's reputation . . . . □ -5

Publisher's reputation . . . . □ -6

Book cover design or layout . . . . □ -7

Index or table of contents of book . . . . □ -8

Price of book . . . . □ -9

Special effects, graphics, illustrations . . . . . . □ -0

Other (Please specify): _____ □ -x

3. How many computer books have you purchased in the last six months? _____ (7-10)

4. On a scale of 1 to 5, where 5 is excellent, 4 is above average, 3 is average, 2 is below average, and 1 is poor, please rate each of the following aspects of this book below. (Please circle your answer.)

Depth/completeness of coverage   5 4 3 2 1   (11)

Organization of material   5 4 3 2 1   (12)

Ease of finding topic   5 4 3 2 1   (13)

Special features/time saving tips   5 4 3 2 1   (14)

Appropriate level of writing   5 4 3 2 1   (15)

Usefulness of table of contents   5 4 3 2 1   (16)

Usefulness of index   5 4 3 2 1   (17)

Usefulness of accompanying disk   5 4 3 2 1   (18)

Usefulness of illustrations/graphics   5 4 3 2 1   (19)

Cover design and attractiveness   5 4 3 2 1   (20)

Overall design and layout of book   5 4 3 2 1   (21)

Overall satisfaction with book   5 4 3 2 1   (22)

5. Which of the following computer publications do you read regularly; that is, 3 out of 4 issues?

Byte . . . . □ -1 (23)

Computer Shopper . . . . □ -2

Corporate Computing . . . . □ -3

Dr. Dobb's Journal . . . . □ -4

LAN Magazine . . . . □ -5

MacWEEK . . . . □ -6

MacUser . . . . □ -7

PC Computing . . . . □ -8

PC Magazine . . . . □ -9

PC WEEK . . . . □ -0

Windows Sources . . . . □ -x

Other (Please specify): _____ □ -y

Please turn page.

6. What is your level of experience with personal computers? With the subject of this book?

	With PCs	With subject of book
Beginner	☐ -1 (24)	☐ -1 (25)
Intermediate	☐ -2	☐ -2
Advanced	☐ -3	☐ -3

7. Which of the following best describes your job title?

Officer (CEO/President/VP/owner)........ ☐ -1 (26)
Director/head............................. ☐ -2
Manager/supervisor....................... ☐ -3
Administration/staff...................... ☐ -4
Teacher/educator/trainer................. ☐ -5
Lawyer/doctor/medical professional....... ☐ -6
Engineer/technician...................... ☐ -7
Consultant............................... ☐ -8
Not employed/student/retired............. ☐ -9
Other (Please specify): _____ ☐ -0

8. What is your age?

Under 20............................... ☐ -1 (27)
21-29.................................. ☐ -2
30-39.................................. ☐ -3
40-49.................................. ☐ -4
50-59.................................. ☐ -5
60 or over............................. ☐ -6

9. Are you:

Male................................... ☐ -1 (28)
Female................................. ☐ -2

Thank you for your assistance with this important information! Please write your address below to receive our free catalog.

Name: _____

Address: _____

City/State/Zip: _____

Fold here to mail.

2397-14-15